CONSCIOUS
CAREGIVING
GUIDE

WISH I KNEW SERIES

CONSCIOUS CAREGIVING GUIDE

WISH I KNEW SERIES

LISE LEBLANC

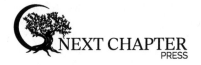

NEXT CHAPTER
PRESS

Wish I Knew: Conscious Caregiving Guide

Editor: Allister Thompson

Book Designer: Jamie Arts

Published in Stratford, Canada, by Blue Moon Publishers.
Printed and bound in Canada.

ISBN: 978-1-988279-91-6

Next Chapter books are available at special quantity discounts to corporations, professional associations and other organizations. For details and discount information, please contact marketing@bluemoonpublishers.com.

CONTENTS

TO MY GRANDMOTHER, EUNICE SOMERS

ABOUT THE WISH I KNEW SERIES:

We create books that help people through life's transitions.

OTHER BOOKS IN THE WISH I KNEW SERIES:

CAREGIVING COLLECTION

Conscious Caregiving Guide
Conscious Caregiving Guide Workbook
Caregiving Insights
Gentle Quotes on Caregiving
Caregiving Guided Journal

GRIEF & LOSS COLLECTION

Conscious Grief & Loss Guide
Conscious Grief & Loss Workbook
Gentle Quotes on Grief & Loss
Grief & Loss Guided Journal

ABOUT THE WISH I KNEW
CAREGIVING COLLECTION

The Wish I Knew Caregiving Collection offers something for every caregiver, whatever stage they are at. Arranged in brief sections, they can be consumed during your caregiving journey, if you only have time to read in a waiting room, while warming up lunch, or during your loved one's nap.

The *Conscious Caregiving Guide* focuses on conscious caregiving and self-care, with brief sections that are broken down with tips, practical exercises, reflective questions, and real-life examples.

The *Conscious Caregiving Guide Workbook* is your essential workbook to accompany the *Conscious Caregiving Guide*. Each chapter in the workbook corresponds to a chapter in the book, including practical exercises, checklists, reflective questions, and more.

Caregiving Insights offers brief stories that offer unique perspectives on caregiving.

Gentle Quotes on Caregiving are brief passages for the harried caregiver who may only have time for a line or two.

The *Caregiving Guided Journal* offers a chance to reflect, recharge, and set aside time for your own self-care.

FOREWORD

Every family has a caregiving story... for better or worse, for richer or poorer, in sickness and in health. Most couples have used just these words as marriage vows promising to provide comfort and care for, "as long as they both shall live".

I'd venture to say, however, that during those tender moments in front of friends and family, neither party gave much thought to what I like to refer to as their "caregiving years". They likely have not discussed how changing circumstances over the years would affect their relationship, their quality of life, their financial situation, their home life and the help they'd have to give or receive.

And can you blame them? Even for those who are not the marrying sort, the topics of retirement planning and financial matters, along with dreams of living somewhere warm, carefree, and affordable usually carry these types of conversations.

Truth is, life happens. Families also drift or fall apart, come back together, blend, change, and grow. Some thrive. Some don't. Regardless, somewhere in our mid to late forties, reality comes knocking for most of us. There's a sibling, a child, a parent, or maybe even a spouse who needs help. And, perhaps, a lot of it. The facts speak for themselves:

More than 8 million Canadians provided informal care to a family member or friend.[1]

More than 1 million caregivers are older than 65.[2]

44% of caregivers between the ages of 45–64 care for both a parent and children.[3]

The number of seniors requiring care is set to double over the next 15 years.[4]

39% of caregivers look after the needs of their parents; 8% care for a spouse.[5]

35% of Canada's workforce provides informal, unpaid care while working.[6]

1.6 million caregivers take time off work to provide care.[7]

One-in-ten caregivers spends more than 30 hours per week providing care.[8]

Caregiving, if we choose to take it on, (and it is a choice), can be a labour of love or a duty depending on who you are. It can be offered hands-on or from afar. It can be full or part time, for a short time or for years. It's a journey through paths unknown that can push a person to their limits and bring out the best or worst in current and past relationships. And no doubt, it's difficult when working, raising a family, going through personal relationship challenges, or raising a child who needs a great deal of extra attention. Yes, looking after someone else can be fraught with financial challenges, emotions, hope, and disappointment. Those who have walked before us will attest to the fact that assuming the role of "carer" it's often referred to these days, is filled with moments of tenderness, kindness, awkwardness, and unfortunately frustration and tribulation.

But, for better or worse, caregiving is simply part of everyday family life for most of us, sooner or later. So, explore the wonderful stories and lessons learned that are shared by experts and laypeople in this book, all with lived experience. I wish you peace, joy, and most of all, increased awareness that will make the time you spend looking after a loved one as stress free, effective, and rewarding as possible for as long as you shall live.

Caroline-Tapp MacDougall

Founder of Canada Cares

Development Manager of Canadian Abilities Foundation

References:
1. Statistics Canada. 2012. "Portrait of Caregivers."
2. Report from the Employer Panel of Caregivers. 2015. "When Work and Caregiving Collide."
3. Ibid.
4. Ibid.
5. Statistics Canada. 2012. "Portrait of Caregivers."
6. Report from the Employer Panel of Caregivers. 2015. "When Work and Caregiving Collide."
7. Ibid.
8. Ibid.

INTRODUCTION

In the movie *What They Had*, actress Ruth Danner plays the role of a wife, mother, and grandmother who has Alzheimer's disease. After she wanders out of the house into a blizzard, the family disagrees about how best to care for her as her illness progresses. Her loving husband wants to do whatever it takes to manage her care at home, while her son who lives close by feels it would be best for her to move into a nursing home. Hilary Swank, who plays her daughter that lives at a distance, is torn between the two. This family's crisis and the challenges, fears, communication problems, emotions, exhaustion, and other complexities they face are commonly experienced by caregivers, including myself. When I suddenly became my grandmother's caregiver, I wanted nothing more than to continue to care for her at home and provide her with the most natural and nurturing environment possible, but I had no idea what I was getting into. I had no idea how deeply challenging this caregiving experience would be. I didn't know if I would have the courage, patience, or commitment to persevere, and I certainly didn't know what I would do if and when the time came where I could no longer care for her.

I was thirty years old, married with two small children when my grand-mother came to live with us. Overnight, I became responsible for providing assistance with shopping, medical appointments, personal hygiene, medica-tion, providing emotional support, and supervision around the clock, seven days per week. I was also coordinating health services and functioning in a legal capacity as her substitute decision-maker. Eventually, I had to advocate for the removal of her driver's license (after two minor accidents and several close calls) and move her into a nursing home for her safety and protection. In all honesty, my grandmother's move to the nursing home was also done in an effort to preserve my own wellbeing. These were not easy decisions, nor were they easy times. Although every caregiving situation is different, I can safely say that no matter how prepared (or unprepared) you may be starting out on your caregiving journey, there will be thoughts, emotions, responsibilities, and situations you will not feel equipped to handle. Like so many other caregivers, I was ill-prepared for the challenges and responsibilities that came with my caregiving role. Unfortunately, I did not handle it nearly as well as I would have liked to, and it took a long time to recover from this experience — mentally, emotionally, physically, and spiritually — but through it all, I learned a lot about what to do (and not to do) as a caregiver. I only *wish I knew* these things when starting my caregiving journey. Therefore, through concrete examples, real-life stories, practical exercises, reflective questions, as well as my personal caregiving journey, this book will provide you with information, insights, and strategies to help you have the best caregiving experience possible. It will answer many of your questions and guide you to enjoy the benefits and rewards of your caregiving relationship while learning to achieve an optimum state of wellness for yourself through it all.

Let me start by sharing how my caregiving journey began...

June 18, 2004

I was packing up and preparing to leave the office on what seemed like a usual Friday afternoon when a colleague showed up at my office door, asking for a favour.

"Is there any chance you could take my on-call duties just for tonight? My daughter is at the hospital with a throat infection."

"Sure, no problem, I have no plans tonight."

"Thanks, I'll pick up the pager first thing in the morning," she said as she dropped the device onto my desk.

She wasn't even out of the building when the pager started beeping. *Are you kidding me?* I thought. I immediately dialled the callback number. Ginette, a front-line case manager, answered and said one of her clients was suicidal and aggressive. We briefly discussed the situation and agreed she should be brought to the hospital for medical evaluation. Trying to find a staff member on a Friday night to come in as backup would be futile, so I headed over to the hospital to meet them. When I arrived, they had already gone through the patient registration process and were sitting in the waiting room. I sat beside the client and gently asked how she was doing. She glanced over and made eye contact for a brief moment before looking back down at the floor. She mumbled in French that she was not doing very well. Her voice was blunt, matching the angry look in her eyes.

"The nurse said it shouldn't be too long," the worker said in a concerned tone. "She will give us the next room that becomes available."

I was relieved to hear we would be able to wait in a private room. There were several people in the general ER waiting room, which I suspected was making the client feel more unsettled. If she did have an aggressive outburst, it would be very difficult to manage, and someone could get hurt.

We made small talk as we waited, but the client's restlessness was palpable. Several more minutes passed when I heard *Code Blue* repeated three times over the loudspeaker. I stood and peeked through the emergency department doors to see paramedics coming in through the back doors with a stretcher. I could hear the commotion and selfishly wondered how much of a delay this person having a heart attack was going to cause.

"This is not good," the worker said, "maybe I should…"

I didn't hear the end of her sentence, because my attention suddenly shifted to the elderly woman rushing frantically through the main entrance doors. She was looking in all directions, confused and disoriented.

"Gramma, what are you doing here?"

"It's Grampa. I think he's dead," she answered frankly.

"*What?*" I figured she had to be mistaken. My grandfather was only seventy-three and in good health. I just saw him the day before. He was completely fine. My grandmother, on the other hand, was not doing so well. Although she was only seventy-two, we had started to notice symptoms of dementia: disorganization, memory loss, and her cognitive abilities were becoming more and more impaired.

I hurried over to the nurses' station with my grandmother in tow. "Excuse me," I interrupted the nurse as she wrote notes on a patient chart.

"You'll have to wait," she replied abruptly without looking up.

"Listen," I said, catching her undivided attention with my firm tone. "My grandfather was brought in on a code blue." Her head snapped up, and her tone instantly softened.

"Oh." She paused for a moment. "Please have a seat in the waiting room. Someone will be out to talk to you very soon."

As we headed back to the waiting room, I tried to get more information from my grandmother. She couldn't tell me much. She was clearly in shock. The only thing she did manage to tell me was that she had called 911 after finding my grandfather unconscious on the bathroom floor.

As we returned to the general waiting area, the worker told me she had already called for backup and had found another manager to take my

14

on-call duties. She asked if there was anything she could do to help. Before I could thank her, I was being summoned back by the nurse. My grandmother followed without saying a word. The nurse greeted us at the emergency room doors and escorted us in.

"Is he going to be okay?" I asked as she guided us to a small private room. She gave me a sympathetic look and told us the doctor would be coming to talk to us soon. Her look said it all.

Shortly after, the doctor arrived. "I'm sorry, we did everything we could," he said with that same sympathetic look. "We are still working on him, but there are no vital signs, and even if we managed to revive him, he has been without oxygen for at least thirty minutes, possibly longer." He turned to my grandmother and asked for her approval to end all life-saving efforts.

She looked at me and said, "I don't know, you decide." The doctor turned to me for an answer. Tears were streaming down my face. I didn't know what to do. From the blank expression on my grandmother's face, I knew she wasn't going to be able to help make this decision. I don't remember what was going through my mind at that exact moment in time, but I do know I did not want to be responsible for making this life-and-death decision.

"Would you like to see him?" the doctor asked.

"Okay," I replied hesitantly, hoping it might help me decide what to do. To this day, I regret not taking the doctor's word for it. I would never be able to unsee what I saw that day: his limp, discoloured body, wires covering his chest, tubes sticking out of his nose, mouth, and arms, his chest covered by medical equipment. As disturbed as I was by the sight of his lifeless body, it instantly made me realize he was really gone, and any further efforts to save his life would be in vain. I knew my grandfather would not want to be kept alive by machines or be disabled and have to rely on someone else for his care. I touched his hand and silently said goodbye before leaving him for the last time.

I had a quick word with my grandmother then let the doctor know that we were in agreement with his recommendation to end all life-saving efforts. I took my grandmother by the hand and walked out through the hospital's main doors into the parking lot. She was in no condition to drive. Come to think of it, neither was I, but I took her keys and helped her into the passenger seat of her car. *What am I going to do with her?* I thought as I slid into the driver's seat. I doubted her ability to live on her own. She was forgetting all kinds of things, like where she put the car keys, how to make favourite recipes, people's names, the date, her address, and where to pick up the mail. At first, I thought it was normal memory loss associated with old age, but recently I'd started noticing other things too. She was always wearing the same clothes, the house wasn't as clean and tidy as it used to be, and she was repeating herself a lot. On several occasions she had cooking mishaps and started doing odd things such as putting spices in the breadbox or ice cream in the cupboard. I was also getting concerned about her driving, because she seemed to be forgetting the rules of the road. When I had tried to talk to my grandfather about it, he reassured me that everything was fine and quickly changed the subject. I had no idea how much he was covering up for her illness, but I was fairly confident she was much worse off than he'd been letting on.

As I drove out of the hospital parking lot, I called my husband, hoping he would know what to do. After giving his condolences and reminding me to call my family, he told me to bring my grandmother to our house for the night. He said we'd figure the rest out in the morning. As I headed to my grandmother's house to get her overnight bag, I called my mom, who lived in Calgary at the time, to tell her that her father had passed on. It turned out to be the toughest call I've ever had to make. I choked back tears as I delivered the bad news. I'd never heard my mom sobbing, and I had no idea how to ease her pain. She wanted to call my Aunt Susan, who lived in Whitehorse, and I agreed to call my sister who lived in London, who then called my Uncle Stan in Chatham. The closest family member lived almost six hours away.

CHAPTER ONE

BECOMING A CAREGIVER

"There are only four kinds of people in the world. Those who have been caregivers. Those who are currently caregivers. Those who will be caregivers, and those who will need a caregiver."

—Rosalyn Carter

Although there are many common caregiving experiences, the roles and responsibilities of caregivers are highly variable. There are so many factors affecting the caregiver role, including: length, degree, complexity and intensity of disability, preparedness and timing of entry into the caregiving role, availability of community resources and family support, relationship dynamics with the care recipient and within the family, as well as shifting roles and responsibilities over time. It also includes degree of disability and prognosis. Is it a permanent disability that will remain stable over time, or one that is expected to deteriorate (e.g., dementia or Parkinson's)? Is the care recipient temporarily disabled and expected to make a partial or full recovery, such as in some stroke and cancer situations? How long will the care recipient be in need of care, and will it get better or worse over time? Will the caregiving role expand and shift as the care recipient becomes increasingly impaired and the illness progresses? So many questions. So many unknowns.

BECOMING A CAREGIVER

Becoming a caregiver can happen in many different ways and can involve several factors, as listed above. Perhaps your spouse has an accident, your parent falls ill, or your child has a disability. Sometimes you take on the responsibilities of caregiving over a long period of time as a loved one's health deteriorates, and other times, as in my situation, it happens unexpectedly and literally overnight. After my grandfather's death, my grandmother's condition deteriorated very rapidly. She had become so dependent on my grandfather that her anxiety increased exponentially, and we quickly realized she could not manage on her own. Although some people are very headstrong and inflexible about receiving care, my grandmother easily recognized and accepted the fact that she was not capable of caring for herself, much less keeping up with the responsibilities of maintaining a large home. She readily agreed to sell her house and came to live with us.

PRACTICAL EXERCISE — HOW YOU BECAME A CAREGIVER

Take a moment to think about how you became a caregiver and write about your story the way I did in the introduction to this book. Try to remain objective and factual in your description, providing as much detail as possible without adding judgements upon yourself or others.

REFLECTIVE QUESTIONS

- How did you initially feel about becoming a caregiver?
- What factors led you to becoming a caregiver?
- In what ways did you feel mentally, emotionally, and physically prepared to become a caregiver at that time in your life? In what ways did you feel unprepared?

CAREGIVING CATEGORIES, TYPES, AND LEVELS OF CARE

Most of us are caregivers in one sense or another at some point in our lives. Some of us choose to become caregivers in our professional lives by selecting professions where we are paid to be caregivers, such as doctors, nurses, personal support workers, therapists, child care workers, etc. Some of us choose to become caregivers in our personal lives, such as when we become parents, or when we take on some or all of the responsibilities of caring for a loved one.

There are so many different types of caregivers, both personally and professionally, but for this purpose I will focus on caregiving in a nonpaid, personal sense, including: 1) caregivers who live with the care recipient; 2) caregivers who live nearby; and 3) caregivers who live far away. Each of these caregiving situations poses different challenges and can include several variables. For example, your care recipient may require a high level of care (full care) or very little care (e.g., check-ins, assistance with medication, or getting to appointments). Additionally, you may be the primary caregiver, a joint-primary caregiver, or a secondary caregiver. My informal definitions for these caregiving categories are as follows:

a. Primary Caregiver: You are the one responsible for providing and coordinating care for your loved one. Everyone knows this and calls upon you when there is a problem, real or perceived. If anything is needed or goes wrong, you are expected to solve the problem. This may have been decided formally through conversations with the care recipient and/or family members, or perhaps it happened informally due to assumptions and/or factors such as you being the oldest, the closest, the most responsible, or due to the nature of your relationship (i.e., a spouse or parent may have a higher level of expectation than a brother or friend, for instance). Or perhaps it was just a matter of you stepping up to the plate before anyone else, and now people are relying on you to continue to carry most of the caregiving responsibilities.

b. Joint-Primary Caregiver: This is a situation when one or more individuals are jointly and relatively equally responsible for the care of a loved one. For example, one of my colleagues was from a large family. As a nurse, the family relied on her for anything related to their semi-independent mother's physical health, such as checking on her in times of sickness, medication side effects, and doctor's appointments. Her sister who was equally involved provided assistance with grocery shopping, meal preparation, and weekly errands. Another sister was responsible for daily phone check-ins, and so on. Their responsibilities were determined in advance based on skill set, availability, and personal preferences. They agreed as much as possible that they would attempt to share the caregiving duties equally.

c. Secondary Caregiver: As a secondary caregiver, you may be consulted to make important decisions or to fill in for specific tasks. You may have regular duties, but they were likely assigned to you by the primary caregiver. As a secondary caregiver, you are not the main person responsible for providing or coordinating care but are providing assistance to the primary caregiver(s).

Within these caregiver categories, there are often caregiver types. You may or may not recognize yourself in one or more of the definitions below:

The Doormat: The person who can't say no. This goes beyond being a kind, decent, and giving human being. The Doormat is "too nice" and tries to please everyone at their own expense. They usually find themselves doing too much and taking on things they really don't want to do, usually leading to resentment and passive-aggressive behaviour.

The Hero: Usually a high achiever both in and out of the home. They are responsible, perfectionists, and master problem-solvers. They can get things done and rarely ask for help. It doesn't matter whether they have the time or energy — the task will get done, and done right! Unlike the doormat, the hero doesn't do it to be nice or because they can't say no. They usually do it because it makes them feel like the special "one" — the one who gets to save the day.

The Martyr: The person who makes huge sacrifices and makes sure everyone knows it. They want everyone to be aware of how much they are doing and how much they are giving up. They often act like the victim and look for pity, praise, or reassurance.

The Sheep: Shies away from everything. They may say they want to help but are never around when it's time to help out. They always have an excuse for not being available.

The Surfer: Is never around. They are off living carefree lives. They might check in once in a while to see how things are going, but their loved one's care is near the bottom of their priority list (hint: if you are the "surfer," you are not reading this book).

The Fighter: Is the one who over-advocates. They are always mad at someone, including doctors, family members, other caregivers, and health-care providers. They pick fights with whoever is around and claim to be acting in the best interest of the care recipient. They have found a sense of purpose and importance in fighting for what's "right," and as such, they can come off as bullies.

The Judge: The person who judges what everyone else is doing or not doing. It can be someone heavily involved in providing care or someone judging from the sidelines. Regardless of where they stand, they can do no wrong, and others can seemingly do no right.

The Helper: May be helping out of the goodness of their heart or out of a sense of obligation. Regardless of their motivations, you can always count on them. They will rarely take on a primary caregiving role but are invaluable as a secondary caregiver.

The Hider: Is very private and often secretive. They act like everything is fine, no matter what is going on in their lives. They may lie or avoid questions to keep others from finding out how bad their situation is. They don't ask for help and often suffer in silence.

The Zen Master: This type of caregiver is in it for the right reasons and not putting a lot of pressure on themselves to be perfect. They are usually doing whatever is required of them with a sense of peace and gratitude, as well as asking and accepting help as needed. This doesn't mean they never feel resentment, frustration, isolation, or other difficult emotions, but they have a good support network in place and use it.

PRACTICAL EXERCISE — EXAMINE YOUR CAREGIVING SITUATION

Identify what type of caregiver you are by circling your answers to the questions below.

Are you a:

a. Caregiver who lives with the care recipient

b. Caregiver who lives near the care recipient

c. Caregiver who lives at a distance

What would best define your caregiving role?

a. Primary caregiver

b. Joint-primary caregiver

c. Secondary caregiver

What would best describe your care recipient's current level of need?

a. Full-care: Completely or mostly dependent for basic needs

b. Partial care: Needs assistance in some areas but independent in other areas

c. Minimal care: Requires some support meeting certain needs.

Circle the caregiver type(s) that best describes you? If you don't know and want to know, ask someone who is close to you who would give you an honest answer.

a. Doormat   b. Hero   c. Martyr   d. Sheep   e. Surfer

f. Judge   g. Fighter   h. Helper   i. Hider   j. Zen Master

REFLECTIVE QUESTIONS

In your ideal world:

- Would you be a caregiver? If so, what type of caregiver would you be for your loved one (primary, joint-primary, or secondary caregiver)?
- What level of care would you be providing (full, partial, minimal, or no care)?
- Would your preference be to live with your care recipient, live nearby, or live far away?

CAREGIVER RESPONSIBILITIES

Sometimes, caregiving starts gradually with a few extra duties and responsibilities such as checking in on a loved one, bringing them to appointments, picking up prescriptions, or helping with laundry as you recognize the care recipient's need for assistance. Over a period of time, you realize you've become a caregiver. In other situations, a sudden plunge into the caregiving role may be a result of a crisis or an unexpected life-threatening diagnosis without any time to prepare or to plan. Caregiving responsibilities may also evolve over time as the care recipient's ability to care for themselves deteriorates. In other words, responsibilities at the beginning of your caregiving journey may be quite different than the responsibilities you end up with as time goes on and your care recipient's needs increase.

Many who become caregivers don't have the training, skills, resources, or energy required to take on the ever-changing responsibilities associated with their new role. It is virtually impossible to compile a complete list of all potential caregiving responsibilities. The following list includes common caregiving responsibilities to help you think about your own caregiving situation and the caregiving responsibilities you've taken on, as well as those you may be facing in the future:

- Personal care: Feeding, bathing, grooming, toileting, dressing, etc.

- Household tasks and chores: Laundry, cleaning, shopping, picking up mail, etc.

- Medical and health: Medication management, support in making and getting to medical appointments, dealing with mobility issues and medical devices, etc.

- Care coordination, advocacy, and problem-solving: Communication with health professionals, secondary caregivers, and other family members.

- Family: Assistance attending family events, communication with family members, handling disagreements, coordinating responsibilities and joint decision-making, etc.

- Supervision: Care recipient may require minimal supervision while engaging in certain tasks such as cooking or personal care, or they may require a high level of supervision if they are exhibiting high-risk behaviour (e.g., wandering, aggression, etc.)

- Social and recreational support: Assistance in staying connected to social networks and attending recreational activities or social events.

- Providing emotional support as care recipient experiences a gamut of emotions such as fear, frustration, anxiety, and perhaps more severe mental or emotional problems such as depression, for example.

- Spiritual: Help care recipient continue with their spiritual practices (going to church, reading scripture, etc.)

- Financial: Money management, paying bills, dealing with banks, insurances, setting up power of attorney for personal care and finances

- End-of-life planning: Wills, funeral arrangements, advanced care planning, etc.

PRACTICAL EXERCISE — EXAMINE YOUR CAREGIVER RESPONSIBILITIES

On a sheet of paper, write down your care recipient's needs. Include every-thing, regardless of how small or insignificant it may seem. Then with a checkmark indicate whether you are mostly responsible for meeting this need. An important first step in making changes (if changes are required) is acknowledging your current reality as a caregiver. In other words, knowing exactly what you are responsible for and understanding the scope of what you are actually doing will help you understand where adjustments to your caregiving situation may be needed.

REFLECTIVE QUESTIONS

- What caregiving responsibilities are most challenging for you? Which are easiest? Why?

- What caregiving responsibilities might you need some help with?

- If you knew then what you know now, would you do anything differently with respect to taking on caregiver responsibilities? If so, what?

CAREGIVER ROLES

Anyone can become a caregiver at any given stage of life. When you became a caregiver, it is likely you already had many roles in life: parent, spouse, aunt, friend, neighbour, volunteer, grandchild, employee, student, etc. With each of these roles comes responsibilities. Adding the role of caregiver to your list and trying to meet someone else's day-to-day needs while maintaining all of your existing roles and responsibilities can be exhausting and overwhelming. In an ideal world, the caregiver would be able to balance everything, but as the care recipient's needs increase over time, it can start to negatively impact other dimensions of the caregiver's life.

PRACTICAL EXERCISE — EXAMINE YOUR ROLES

Separate a sheet of paper into two columns. In the left-hand column, make a list of all of your roles, both personally and professionally. In the right-hand column, write down as many of the responsibilities you can think of associated with each role. For example, the role of a sister may involve a phone call once a week and a visit once a month, but parenting a young child would include many more duties.

REFLECTIVE QUESTIONS

- What roles did you already have when you became a caregiver?
- What role/relationship did you have with the care recipient prior to them being in need of care?
- Did you feel capable of taking on the added role of being a caregiver?

STRESS AND EMOTIONAL CAPACITY

The time when our loved ones get sick and are no longer able to care for themselves is not our choice. It just happens when it happens. It can be when we are looking forward to an empty nest or excited about retirement plans. Perhaps it happens when we are in the prime of building our lives. When we are busy balancing our own families, careers, finances, and running our households. When our time is already stretched thin, and we're running the rat race, trying to get ahead ... and then BAM! Someone is in need of our care.

When I became my grandmother's caregiver, my son was five and my daughter had just turned one. I had recently completed my master's degree while working full-time as a manager in an agency that was in the process of unionizing. I was also struggling within myself about my abilities as a wife and mother. Needless to say, I was already under extreme stress trying to balance my busy personal life with work and school when my caregiving responsibilities fell into my lap.

Even if you willingly choose to take on the caregiving role, you may quickly realize that you just don't have enough hours in the day or enough mental and emotional resources to get the job done, and there's more on this in Chapter Five — Caregiver Burnout.

PRACTICAL EXERCISE

Divide a sheet of paper into two columns. In the left column, write down all of the extra responsibilities you have taken on as part of your caregiving role. In the right column, place a checkmark beside those you feel stressed about. In your journal, write about how you've been affected by the added stress of becoming a caregiver.

REFLECTIVE QUESTIONS

- What was going on in your life at the time you took on the role and responsibilities of caregiving?
- On a scale of 1 to 5 (1 being low-stress and 5 being high-stress), how would you rate your stress level before becoming a caregiver?
- On a scale of 1 to 5, how would you rate your stress level six months after becoming a caregiver?

RESPITE AND RESOURCES

Perhaps, like me, you are already run-down, without an extra ounce of energy to take on your new role and added responsibilities, or perhaps you're starting out full of energy, thinking it won't be too hard. Regardless of where you're at, your life will be dramatically altered when you become a caregiver, and it will involve many adjustments. The extra responsibilities associated with taking care of someone can be heavy, and other people in your life may not appreciate all that you're doing. In fact, they may not fully realize the actual scope of your contributions or how much mental, emotional, and physical resources are required from you. For this reason, it is very important to put a care plan in place.

Regardless of how strong you may be now or how in control of your life you may think you are, it takes a good support system to be a good caregiver, especially if it is going to be a long-term situation. Sure, you can take on all of the responsibilities and do it on your own for a while, but eventually it will catch up to you. If you're reading this book, you are likely already in some type of caregiving situation, and it is important to acknowledge the toll caregiving might be taking on you. Perhaps your ego is getting in the way of asking for help. Maybe you're worried about what others will think. Maybe you don't want anyone to think you are weak or can't handle it. Or it may be that your care recipient doesn't want to accept help from anyone other than you. However, if you are caregiving beyond your capabilities, over time it will wear you down, and it will not be a healthy situation for you or for your care recipient. Therefore, once you have a care plan in place, take the time to really look at what other resources might be available if and when you and/or your care recipient need them.

PRACTICAL EXERCISE — SET UP A CARE PLAN

Your specific task is to get a few of your close family members and/or friends together, along with your care recipient if possible, to look at your role and responsibilities and develop a plan that outlines your loved one's care needs and determines who will meet those needs and when. Perhaps you are thinking this is *my* daughter or *my* husband, and I am solely responsible for caring for them, but trust me when I say that the full load of caregiver responsibilities can be intense and can put you at very high-risk for burnout. Before the end of this planning meeting, create a schedule and clear expectations about who will be doing what. Be specific and include the task, which days it will be completed, and by whom. Make a copy for everyone, and barring emergencies, stick to the care plan. Allow others to contribute and see if you can create either a "joint-primary care" arrangement where there is a more equal distribution of the responsibilities, or at least set yourself up with several secondary caregivers to assist with your loved one's needs. Keep the list of tasks that remain your responsibility close by in the event someone else asks if or how they can help. Show them the list and discuss if there is anything they might be interested in taking on, either regularly or as a one-time thing. Use the Caregiver Checklist (Appendix A) to help set up your care plan.

REFLECTIVE QUESTIONS

- Who could help with your care recipient's needs: physical, emotional, spiritual, financial, medical?

- When and in what ways are you inviting and allowing others to get involved in your loved one's care?

- If you wanted to, could you do a better job sharing and distributing caregiving duties? If so, how committed are you to developing a care plan for this purpose?

PLANNING

Obviously, I hadn't planned on becoming a caregiver at that time in my life, and I was not set up for it. It wasn't like when we decided to have kids and actually prepared for the responsibility of caring for them; we read books, lined up support from family and friends, organized daycare and babysitters, set up a baby room, bought tiny clothing, bottles, and toys, and tried to anticipate all of the challenges involved in our new role as parents. We talked about how we would continue to carve out time for ourselves as individuals and as a couple. But for some reason, we had no plan for the situation we suddenly found ourselves in, despite the fact that there are millions of people in North America who are part of the "sandwich generation" — the generation simultaneously raising their children and caring for their aging parents, often while working full-time jobs and leading busy social lives. When we become parents, it is usually by choice at a relative time of our choosing. Of course, there are surprises or situations where things aren't quite planned, but with parenting, at least we have nine months to anticipate the challenges, responsibilities, and sacrifices involved. Not everyone chooses to become a parent, but for those of us who do, we had time to prepare for this major life-changing event, whereas becoming a caregiver for a sick or disabled loved one can happen at any point in our lives, whether we're ready or not.

My mom always told me she would end her life before becoming a burden on anyone. Although I don't like her plan and would much rather assist in her care, she is adamant about this, so I never really gave much thought to the possibility of becoming a caregiver on a personal level other than to take care of my own kids. But here I was.

The fact that we are *all* very likely to become a caregiver at some point in our lives, beyond caring for our own children, does beg the question of why we don't plan in advance for these situations. Sure, some people die suddenly and never need a day of care in their lives, as in my grandfather's case. Perhaps this is what we all aspire to, but in reality, many of us will develop chronic illnesses and require care. Considering the fact that most of us will at one time or another be a caregiver or a care recipient, why is it we don't do a better job preparing for this nearly inevitable situation?

PRACTICAL EXERCISE — GET ORGANIZED

Perhaps your care recipient is partially independent and still able to do many things on their own, or maybe they are already at a point where they need a high level of care. Regardless of their current needs and abilities, unless your care recipient is expected to make a full and speedy recovery, I would strongly suggest you start planning and preparing for their future needs. Use the Caregiver Checklist (Appendix A) to help with your planning efforts. Completing this exercise will give you peace of mind, knowing that you are organized, on top of things, and ready for what may lie ahead.

REFLECTIVE QUESTIONS:

- Do you have a good handle on your care recipient's medical information?

- Are you organized with respect to your care recipient's financial future?

- How have you prepared for emergencies related to your caregiving situation?

CONCLUSION

It is easy to become overwhelmed as a caregiver, and taking an honest look at your caregiving role and responsibilities is an important first step in getting back on track. Setting realistic expectations and accepting help can go a long way in keeping you healthy and well on your caregiving journey. If you haven't already done so, take the time to identify all of the secondary caregivers. Include anyone who is checking in, asking questions, and showing concern. Make a list of all of the resources available in your community for caring for your loved one, as well as caring for yourself. Examine whether there are additional resources you haven't tapped into yet. Putting this work in at the front end might seem like too much effort, but this is what will save you in the long run. It is a huge mistake to forget about yourself and what *you* want and need. Sometimes the greatest gift you can give a loved one is to show them you are still able to enjoy your life to the fullest while caring for them. When your loved one sees you prioritizing your own health and your own needs, it may ease their mind and their guilt about being a burden on you. So many times we think we have to sacrifice ourselves for our loved ones, but what if we can continue living our lives to the fullest while still finding creative ways to meet their care needs?

CHAPTER TWO

CAREGIVER EMOTIONS

"Relationships based on obligation lack dignity."

—Wayne Dyer

Perhaps you are in a chapter of life where you can embrace your situation and enjoy the humble calmness of walking a difficult journey with a loved one. If this is you, commend yourself for being one of the rare few for whom the caregiving experience comes at the right time in your life and for the right reasons. I would venture to say that for most, although we would love to embrace our caregiving experience with joy, love, patience, and gratitude, we are not so fortunate.

Timing, circumstances, and capacity play an important role in how you feel about being a caregiver. If you chose to become a caregiver at a good time in your life and feel confident in your ability to provide care, you are likely experiencing more joy, gratitude, fulfillment, connection, and personal growth and less of the difficult emotions — or at least not experiencing them as frequently or as intensely. When I went through my own caregiving experience, I had certain emotional challenges that no one seemed to be talking about. I wasn't experiencing the sense of purpose and personal satisfaction that I perceived others were feeling. What was wrong with me? My grandmother had been one of the most important and loving caregivers in my life, and when she got ill, I felt stuck, burdened, and resentful. I could not care for her in the loving playful way that she'd cared for me. Instead I felt impatience, frustration, and a whole host of negative emotions. I didn't want to feel this way and felt terribly guilty about it. If you find yourself frustrated, anxious, angry, losing patience, and/

or exhausted, understand it is a common experience, but it also signals a time to honestly reflect on your situation and consider making changes to benefit both your care recipient and yourself.

Although it is impossible to cover every emotion caregivers experience (or how they may experience them), I will touch on those I personally struggled with, as well as those I have heard about most often from other caregivers. Since there is such a wide range of emotions, with considerable overlap, I have grouped similar emotions together for the purpose of addressing as many emotions as possible.

EMOTIONAL ROLLER COASTER

I can appreciate many people have good caregiving experiences that include a mix of both negative and positive emotions. While I do believe there are many benefits and rewards to caregiving, I also believe it is important to talk about the not-so-positive aspects. Since my own caregiving experience, I have heard many caregiving stories, both personally and professionally, and I now know that I was not alone in experiencing serious emotional challenges as a caregiver. Many have described the experience as an emotional roller coaster filled with highs and lows, as well as unexpected twists and turns. Sometimes you're laughing, sometimes crying, other times you feel dizzy and disoriented and just want to get off. Several caregivers have admitted to me that even when they were talking about how great it was to be blessed with this opportunity to care for their elderly mother, or ill husband, or disabled child, there were parts of the experience that were not easy and not pleasant.

PRACTICAL EXERCISE — IDENTIFY YOUR EMOTIONS

Separate a sheet of paper in two. In the left column, make a list of the positive emotions you are experiencing as part of your caregiving journey. In the right column, make a list of all of your negative emotions. Once your list is complete, rate on a scale of 1 to 5 how intensely you are experiencing each emotion (1 being least intense and 5 being most intense).

REFLECTIVE QUESTIONS

- Do you feel like you are on an emotional roller coaster? If so, journal about the emotional ride you've been on.
- What have been the best aspects of caregiving?
- What have been the worst aspects of caregiving?

OBLIGATION AND BURDEN

When my grandmother came to live with us, I did not feel capable of taking on this added responsibility, but it was the only viable option we could come up with. She did not want to live in a nursing home, and I was the only family member who lived close by. Not only did I feel a tremendous sense of responsibility, but I also felt a huge amount of obligation to take on the responsibility of her care. My grandmother had been one of my most loving caregivers when I was a child. I loved her very much and was extremely grateful for all that she gave me. I sometimes think I would not be where I am today if it wasn't for her unconditional love and care. I owed her. At least that's how it felt. I didn't know how I was going to do it, but it was my duty, and I couldn't let her or my family down. With everyone so far away, the burden was all mine.

For some, the caretaker role is taken on consciously and wholeheartedly, and for others, it is done grudgingly. Although no one actually coerced me into taking on this role, I didn't feel like anyone was considering the time, energy, or other burdens it was placing on me and my family. It certainly was not the dream life we wanted, and it felt as though I was giving up my life, or at least significant parts of it. My sense of obligation was very much driving my motivation for caregiving.

This begs the question: *Is caregiving an act of love or of obligation?* And the answer is ... it depends. For my grandmother caring for her grandchildren, I believe it was very much an act of love. For me, it was mainly motivated by a sense of obligation. For others it is both. Also, it can start as an act of love and turn into obligation, or vice versa. Both in my personal and professional capacities, I have come across many people who have experienced the caregiving role in one way or another along this continuum. The experience is different for everyone. To illustrate, here are some things other caregivers have said about their experiences:

"This may sound strange, but becoming my wife's caregiver makes me feel needed. My wife used to take care of me, the kids, and the household. Sometimes I felt like she didn't need me at all, because she did everything on her own and didn't seem to want help. But since her illness, I've been taking care of her and participating a lot more with the kids and the chores.

Sometimes I feel like it's too much and get overwhelmed, but most of the time, it has given me a sense of purpose, and I feel more connected to her than ever."

"For me it was an obligation, and I felt like I put my life on hold for six years. As much as I hate to admit it, I'm glad it's over."

"My daughter was born with severe mental and physical disabilities. I love her with every fibre of my being, and every day I thank God for the blessings she has brought to my life. It doesn't mean I don't get tired at times, but overall I am happy to dedicate my life to caring for her."

"My son has brain damage because of an overdose. I have been taking care of him and helping support his two kids. I resent him for the situation he's put me in."

"Caregiving for my husband in his time of need is a gift, but I do miss what we had before. With his cognitive impairments, we can no longer have the intellectual conversations we used to. In some ways, I don't really feel like his wife anymore, and it can be very lonely at times."

"I've been a caregiver my whole life, and I'm sick and tired of it. I feel trapped, and I feel like screaming. I don't even want to get out of bed in the morning."

"I can't think too much about all of the things I gave up to care for my aging mother, because if I do, I get very sad. I chose to do this out of love but am starting to wonder if it was the right choice."

"I started my caregiving duties with love and gratitude, but now after two years I am exhausted. I hope someday I will look back on this experience and feel like it was the right thing to do."

"I love caring for others, but I need a break from it. Now that I'm in it, I don't know how to get out of my commitments."

"For me caregiving is what I do. I don't know who I'd be or what I would do if I was not a caregiver. Perhaps I need to be needed. I don't know. But I do know that I get a huge sense of personal satisfaction and joy out of helping others. First, I provided care for my disabled son, then my husband developed a mental illness, and now I am caring for my mother who has Alzheimer's disease. Sometimes it's hard, but it brings purpose and meaning to my life."

"I'm lonely, tired, scared, anxious, stuck, and afraid that at any moment another shoe will drop and he will need even more care than he does now ... or worse. I feel guilty that I want and need to have something other than this — challenging work, travel, time with my grandkids ... a future."

As you can see from these quotes, caregiving can come from a place of love and be very fulfilling. It can also be something we're doing out of a sense of obligation. For most, I believe it's both — loving and rewarding *and* a burden and obligation.

PRACTICAL EXERCISE — LOVE AND/OR OBLIGATION?

Take some time to think about how you truly feel about caregiving. Journal about it and then destroy the pages you wrote on. Knowing no one will ever see what you wrote may allow you to be more honest than you've ever been about your feelings as a caregiver.

REFLECTIVE QUESTIONS

Take a look at your different caregiver roles, both personally and professionally, and for each caregiver role, answer the following questions:

- Was this caregiver role taken on as a real choice? For every role you answered that was a choice, indicate on a scale of 1 to 5 the level of choice (1 being that it was not a choice at all and 5 being that it was fully a choice).

- What have been the rewards and costs of your caregiving experiences when it was a choice? What have been the rewards and costs of your caregiving experiences when it did not feel like a choice?

- What differences have you noticed between the caregiver roles you chose versus those you felt forced into?

GUILT AND SHAME

Author Tia Walker wrote, "To care for those who once cared for us is one of the highest honours." As much as I would like to believe I am a good enough person to embrace this quote, I highly dislike it, because when it came time to care for my grandmother, I did not want to. This brought a lot of guilt and shame, because I had no desire to change my life to care for her, despite the fact that she had cared for me so selflessly. It became something I had to do, and it led to resentment, anger, feeling stuck and burdened, as well as many other difficult feelings. Perhaps the most difficult was guilt and shame. The meaning I attached to it was what made it so shameful. For me, it basically meant I was *a bad person* for not wanting to make the sacrifices to care for her and repay my debt, so to speak. I have since realized my grandmother never thought of caring for me as a sacrifice. It was not forced on her at a bad time in her life. It was her choice and her desire. My Gramma did not expect or want me to sacrifice myself for her.

Guilt comes in many forms. Sometimes it is feeling bad for enjoying a night out with friends while your bedridden spouse is being cared for by a volunteer, or your disabled child is being babysat by a neighbour, or perhaps you feel guilty simply because you are still able to enjoy your life while they are incapacitated. Sometimes guilt comes from thinking you should be doing more or should have done something differently. Maybe you feel guilty for getting angry at your loved one or doing something you wish you hadn't done. You might be feeling guilty because feelings of resentment or negative thoughts have built up. There are too many sources of guilt to name, but what is most important in all of this is understanding that every caregiver feels guilt for one thing or another at some point on their caregiving journey. Instead of beating yourself up, put that energy to good use and start looking at more productive ways to transform feelings of guilt into something more positive and productive.

PRACTICAL EXERCISE — GUILT AUDIT

For the next few days, conduct a "guilt audit" by keeping a journal and record-ing each incident in which you catch yourself feeling guilty. Write down the factors that lead to you feeling guilty, as well as the thoughts that are keeping the guilt alive.

REFLECTIVE QUESTIONS

Using a recent incident from your guilt audit, ask yourself the following questions:

- If you could go back and do things differently, what would you change? Although there is no rewind or delete button, sometimes the best thing we can do is learn from past actions what didn't work so well and then commit to doing better next time.

- Instead of berating yourself, is there anything you can say or do to set things right within yourself or with someone else (if others were involved)?

- Could you let this go if you really wanted to? For example, if someone were to offer you $5,000 to let it go, could you? What would need to happen for you to let this go?

RESENTMENT, ANGER, AND FRUSTRATION

Even if you love the person you are caring for, when you are a caregiver, resentment is bound to build. Frustration is almost inevitable. We cannot be everything to everyone, so even with the best intentions, even with the best attitude, you may not be able to fulfill your caregiver duties with complete joy and willingness. You may get angry. At times you may feel like you are on your last nerve, and there may even be times when you totally lose it. Even when acting out of the goodness of our hearts, there is only so much we can handle. Only so much we want to handle. When taking on more than we really want to, the extra burden may turn to resentment, anger, and frustration. These feelings may come across as impatience or negative judgements. You may find yourself correcting your loved one, rushing them, snatching things from them, or even losing your temper with them. You may yell or say something hurtful or perhaps have bad thoughts about them. You might even wish for them to be gone.

A lack of resentment, on the other hand, looks calm, natural, and relaxed. It looks like a grandmother playfully interacting with a grandchild. It looks like patience, kindness, and love.

In my opinion and experience, as well as through information gathered from many other caregivers, occasional feelings of anger, resentment, and frustration are a very normal part of the caregiving experience. Experiencing these thoughts and feelings can even be a positive thing, as in the caregiving example below, where a care recipient talks about the frustrations that arise between her and her husband and how voicing these feelings can sometimes lead to more constructive outcomes and deeper understandings.

> There are times when anger rears its ugly head. As we move through different stages of my illness, there are times of anger and frustration. And it is on both of our parts. I have lashed out at him when he didn't deserve it because something was triggered or hurting inside of me. Something that had to do with my own stuff and nothing to do with him. Other times, he's reached a point of frustration with my situation. A point where he has no idea how to help or how to deal with it. There are rare

times when he gets mad and says things like, "I can't deal with this. I can't come home from my day and deal with your issues." These moments are very painful and difficult to navigate, and yet they sometimes elicit the most authentic truths. Truths that are painful at the time. Truths that take us away from each other for a while. But truths that ultimately bring us closer together and lead to a more intimate understanding and acceptance of each other. It allows us to heal hurts and move forward with a new awareness and a new appreciation for each other.

If you are having angry thoughts and feelings, it does not mean you should not be a caregiver. However, if you're predominantly feeling resentful, angry, and frustrated, then it is time to dig deep within yourself and think about making positive changes to your caregiving situation.

PRACTICAL EXERCISE — IDENTIFY YOUR RESENTMENTS

Resentment usually surfaces when we feel undervalued and unappreciated. Built-up resentment leads to anger and frustration. Thinking about your caregiving experience, make a list of all things you are angry, hurt, or upset about. Start at the beginning of your caregiving journey and be very thorough. It can be helpful to work through this in small increments of time (such as six-month periods).

REFLECTIVE QUESTIONS

- For each of these events on your list, indicate why you are resentful.
- How have you been affected by each of the incidents?
- What have you done, if anything, to clear out your resentments?

FEAR AND ANXIETY

What if something goes wrong? Am I responsible? How will I cope? Caregivers often have fears about what might happen and how they will handle all of the "what-ifs." Sometimes our fears involve what is happening right now and are easily solvable, but many fears are more of a deep-rooted nature. Fears can be numerous, including but not limited to: fear of incompetence; fear of change; fear of responsibility; fear of what we are losing; fear of judgement, by others and/or ourselves; fear of being a "bad" person if we say no; fear of hurting someone who has loved us for so long; and fear of not being able to (or wanting to) deal with an illness or the needs and demands of our care recipient. It's important to remember that these fears come from somewhere, and the source is often not obvious until we start to untangle our own story. Here is a concrete example of my own deep-rooted fears through a partial transcript of one of my therapy sessions during the time I was experiencing caregiver burnout (more on this in Chapter Five):

> "You're not the only option here. Let someone else take care of her," my counsellor challenged.

> "What do you mean there are other options? Do you see anyone else here?"

> "Why would anyone else disrupt their lives, or even know that you need help when you've got everything under control," he continued.

> "I can't put that on them. They all live far away."

> "So what?" he challenged further.

> I was speechless, which doesn't happen often.

> "Lise, you are not responsible for your grandmother. You need to get that."

> "I'm all she's got. She took care of me my whole life. I can't just leave her to fend for herself and hope someone will come to the rescue. What am I supposed to do?"

"Well, why don't you start by getting honest with your family? Why don't you let them know how your health and well-being are being affected by this? Maybe it's time to let them know you're heading for a burnout. Or already there."

"I don't want to tell my family that I've failed them. That I've failed her."

"Why did you take this on anyway?" he pressured relentlessly.

"I just told you, there's no one else!" I said, my tone getting louder.

"I don't think I've heard the real reason yet. Tell me ... why do you see yourself as a failure if you can't do this?"

My anger suddenly turned to tears as I went on to explain how I'd been the black sheep of the family and how this was the first time I felt like I had any value to them. This ah-ha moment made me realize that there was a lot more affecting my emotional state than the responsibilities I had taken on. My worth as a human being, my value to my family was in question. I was afraid they wouldn't love or value me if couldn't succeed at this.

He continued, "When you learn to reach out to the people who matter to you and tell them you're scared, confused, discouraged, hurt, pissed off, and be vulnerable to the thoughts and feelings you're having, this is when things will start to turn around for you. You need to talk to your family and let them know how you're feeling and where you're at. I don't know your family. In fact, I know nothing about them, but I'm going to venture a guess that if they knew what you're telling me, they would find other options for your grandmother's care."

"I just feel like I'm failing everyone ... once again I'll be the family fuck-up."

"You need to get out of this story of failure. This is just another story that's feeding your fear and preventing you from doing what's right for you ... and probably what's best for your grandmother."

I was afraid of being the family failure, which led me to becoming the family "hero." Your fears may be much different than mine. This is simply one example of how our deep-rooted fears can keep us from doing the right thing for our own well-being as well as for the well-being of our care recipient. When I did come clean to my family, they did not judge me as a failure at all. In fact, I got quite the opposite reaction. They immediately banded together to find solutions. They also apologized for not realizing how hard this had been on me. Even if their reaction would have reinforced my failure story, it is important to understand how our fears rooted in past experiences can keep us stuck and blind us from potential solutions that are right in front of us.

PRACTICAL EXERCISE — IDENTIFY YOUR DEEP-ROOTED FEARS

Without even realizing it, deep-rooted fears may be controlling you, your life, your relationships, and your decision-making. These fears are almost always taken on very early in life and can be very powerful. Take the time to reflect on the source of your fears and to look at where they came from. If you are unable to identify the root of your fear, it will be nearly impossible to overcome it.

REFLECTIVE QUESTIONS

- What are you afraid will happen if you get honest with yourself and with others about your caregiving challenges?
- What are you worried you will be judged about?
- What would you do differently in your caregiving situation if you weren't stuck in fear?

UNCERTAINTY, UNPREDICTABILITY, AND THE UNKNOWN

Most of us want to feel like we are in the driver's seat. We want to feel like we are in control, we have a plan, and life is predictable. We want to think we know what's going to happen. Yet so much of our caregiving experience is out of our control, and this state of uncertainty can be very hard to handle. We all need to understand that "NOW" is the only moment we really have. The rest lies in uncertainty, even in those times when we believe our future is certain. Here's Jane's story as an example to illustrate how unpredictability and the unknown are very much a part of the journey as a caregiver.

When Bob and I got married, we made a conscious decision not to include the "in sickness and in health" and "'til death do us part" portion of the traditional wedding vows. They had been words we both spoke at our previous weddings that hadn't been honoured. We decided to be together and felt it would always be our choice to stay together. We discussed the age difference (he is thirteen years older than I am) and the fact that he had a distinct genetic propensity to significant vision and cardiac issues. We'd be fine, we said, nothing we couldn't cope with. We didn't see cancer, hemodialysis, and dementia in his future.

Bob is entering his seventh year of dialysis, a life-sustaining medical procedure that requires fifteen hours per week at the hospital, diet and fluid restrictions, and extra sleep. His cancer has recurred after almost eight years, is stable for now, but it hovers in the background. His cognitive problems have progressed from mild memory loss and intermittent word-finding issues to severe loss of short-term memory, difficulty following conversations, problem-solving, and challenges with some elements of day-to-day activities. To look at him or talk to him briefly, you wouldn't think anything was wrong. As he says himself, *I look fine on the outside, but not so good on the inside.* However, much to his chagrin, his issues are becoming more obvious on the outside as well.

Our life consists mostly of dialysis, medical appointments, reminders to take meds, repetition of "what's up today?", the gradual handoff of activities he used to do and enjoy (i.e., cooking), and withdrawal from social situations. He still argues with me at times that he doesn't have dementia, "he could drive if he wanted to, no problem," and "so what if I don't know what day it is." He is becoming much more negative, complaining that "nobody tells me anything" and "the damn remote won't work right." He used to be very upbeat and optimistic. We used to laugh so much, and still do sometimes, but for the most part life just isn't that fun or funny anymore.

We both know that this isn't going to end well. We have discussed and planned for his end of life, his funeral. Heck, he even designed his tombstone, and it sits waiting for him at the family plot. The average life span of a dialysis patient is around five to ten years. The cancer and heart issues negatively influence that prognosis. The dementia likely isn't life-threatening, it just makes life more problematic.

While we can still rationally discuss things, we agree that we have to do what works for both of us. He doesn't want to hold me back. He understands that it isn't much fun sitting around watching him sleep. He is open to options, and we are actively exploring alternatives. There are many things to consider and a key question: how do you plan when so much is uncertain? Every day is different, some better than others. Each medical test increases our anxiety. This journey could end next month, or it could go on for several more years. His care needs could increase dramatically. We could be facing a decision to continue or stop dialysis. I could get sick myself and be unable to look after him. We don't know how this will play out. We are struggling to figure it out. My caregiver journey continues indefinitely, and I hope I can continue to cope. For now, we sit in limbo. We wait. We wonder.

PRACTICAL EXERCISE — COPING WITH UNCERTAINTY

Journal about how you have been coping with uncertainty. Write about how you handle changing situations, unpredictability, and the unknown.

REFLECTIVE QUESTIONS

- How can you let go of control and learn to live in the moment? Think of at least three things you could let go of if you really wanted to.

- How would your life be different if you practiced living in the moment?

- Can you accept "what is" if things in your life were to stay exactly as they are for another five years or more?

HOPELESSNESS, DESPAIR, AND DEPRESSION

Recently, I met a woman who told me about the hopelessness and despair she feels on her caregiving journey. She has an eight-year-old daughter with many cognitive and physical impairments. She does not communicate, is not toilet-trained, and requires twenty-four-hour supervision. Mom is very dedicated to her daughter's care but has very little support. Dad is in the picture but provides only minimal care every other weekend. She has a wonderful neighbour who pitches in when she can, but it's nowhere near what she needs to manage her daughter's illness, which requires several trips to the hospital, medication management, total personal care, constant supervision, and so much more. Her daughter's care will be a life-long commitment. There will be no independence, ever. Most times, Mom is okay with this, but then there are the late-night conversations with herself. The ones fraught with hopelessness. Feelings of despair and sometimes the desire to escape her life, at least for a little while. With no finish line in sight and no hope that the situation will ever get better, the responsibilities, even though she wouldn't change it for the world, are overwhelming and even depressing at times.

It is not unusual for caregivers to develop symptoms of depression as a result of dealing with a difficult situation over extended periods of time, often while sacrificing their own needs. The various demands of the caregiver role can strain even the most competent and capable person. However, people who take an active, problem-solving approach to caregiving are less likely to feel helpless, hopeless, and depressed and are more likely to realize the positive benefits of caregiving. However, this is one of those things that can be easier said than done, as you can see from the words of a woman who is currently going through the caregiving journey:

> Intellectually, I know what I need to do; ask for help more than I do, be honest with friends and family about what is happening and what both of us need, figure out a way to maintain my life so I can carry on after this is all over, ignore what I perceive as other people's judgments about how we are managing and not get so hung up on anticipating worst-case scenarios. Look

for things to be grateful for each day, find joy where we can, be happy my husband is still here with me, meditate, and take long walks. But practically, I have always had trouble implementing the theory.

One thing that can really help is to join a caregiver support group. This is a safe place to say the unspeakable out loud with people who are going through their versions of the caregiver experience. It's an opportunity to talk about what's affecting you, to give and get support from people who 'get it' and to share information about community resources. Trust me, if you haven't already realized this, you will eventually come to terms with the fact that trying to do this alone is a very lonely and isolating experience, which can lead to hopelessness, despair, and depression.

PRACTICAL EXERCISE — JOIN A SUPPORT GROUP

Find a local support group in your community and go to a meeting this week. If you can find a support group specific to your caregiving situation, great! If not, join a general caregiving support group and start learning how to maximize the resources available to you.

REFLECTIVE QUESTIONS

- Do you regularly feel joy, gratitude, and a general sense of contentment? If not, look at what is preventing you from achieving this state of being? List at least five factors.
- How often do you feel hopeless, helpless, overwhelmed, trapped, and exhausted? What specific action steps could you take to feel less hopeless and more joyful?
- Has anyone suggested the need to take better care of yourself? If so, have you taken their suggestions?

CONCLUSION

Emotions are part of being human, and caregiving can be a particularly emotional journey, but this does not mean we have to be slaves to our emotions. We must recognize and accept our feelings of resentment, frustration, anger, fear, guilt, hopelessness, loneliness, shame, etc., and examine where these feelings are coming from. We need to allow ourselves to feel them, because they are authentic. Everyone has them, but not everyone has the vulnerability and courage to admit it. One thing I have learned through my caregiving experience is that guilt, helplessness, resentment, and other negative emotions do not create good energy for the caregiver or the care recipient. We sometimes forget the value of positive energy and the importance of honouring our emotions. As mentioned previously, caregiving can be very rewarding, but for most it is also very challenging. It requires a lot of time, energy, and hard work, and if you don't pay attention to your own needs and emotions, you are potentially damaging the relationships that matter to you most, including your relationship with yourself.

CHAPTER THREE

CAREGIVING RELATIONSHIPS

"Connection is why we're here;
it is what gives purpose and
meaning to our lives."

—Brené Brown

Relationships can be complicated in the best of times, and when your loved one is affected by a serious illness or disability, it can complicate the relationship that much more. So how do we navigate this world of relationships when we suddenly find ourselves in a situation we didn't want or expect? Whether your spouse can no longer work, do chores, participate in routine activities, or provide mental or emotional support due to illness, or your child is born with a life-long disability, or your elderly parent can no longer care for themselves, the vision you had for your future, and theirs, is crushed. Life as you know it and expected it to be is lost. As roles and relationships are redefined, it is normal and natural for this to have an impact on your level of happiness and sense of fulfillment. As much as you want to have a healthier, more connected relationship with your care recipient, you must first understand that you are responsible for your own happiness. We can easily put the burden on others to make us happy, or blame them for our lack of happiness, but the best thing you can do for any relationship (and for yourself) is learn to love yourself, be responsible for your own needs, and live in accordance with your values.

REDEFINING RELATIONSHIPS

Perhaps your situation is one where your caregiver role started on day one of the relationship, such as with the birth of a child with a disability. Or perhaps when your loved one got sick, your relationship completely shifted from what it used to be. Either way, the relationship you thought you were going to have was redefined. For example, if your parent has dementia, you may find yourself in a role reversal where you are acting like the parent, and your parent becomes more like the child in the relationship. If your spouse lost his ability to care for his physical needs, you may feel more like his nurse than his wife. This can put great strain on the relationship and change the entire dynamic.

While everyone is different and every relationship has its unique aspects, there are some common experiences. Here are a few anonymous quotes to illustrate some of the changes in relationship roles and dynamics that can be experienced:

> "I have become the caregiver, the driver, the nurse, the decision-maker, the house manager, and not so much the wife anymore. The nature of our relationship has changed from a true partnership between independent adults to one that more closely resembles a parent-child relationship."

> "When my mother developed Alzheimer's disease, her whole personality changed. She became angry and abusive. I could no longer go to her for advice or emotional support. She went from being my rock to a cement block tied to my ankle in a pool of water. I never imagined this would be our relationship."

> "Since my husband's stroke, I do all of the household duties like grocery shopping, cooking, and laundry, plus I now have to cut the grass, take out the garbage, and do all the things that I never had to do before. Now, I do my stuff, the stuff he used to be in charge of, plus I have to take care of him. My role has expanded so much that I don't even know who I am anymore ... as a person or as a wife. My whole identity has been shattered by this."

> "My mother went from being my best friend, the babysitter for my son, the person that took care of family gatherings and someone I could always rely on, to someone who absolutely drains the life out of me."

> "When my daughter was born with cerebral palsy and I was told she would likely never walk or talk, I selfishly felt like my

life was over. Not only would I never see her grow up into a healthy, independent adult, but I would forever be responsible for her care. It took me a while before I could finally face my new reality."

In one situation, a husband told me that no matter how dire or permanent his wife's deteriorating health situation was, he could not let go of the hope that she would miraculously get better one day. He saw it as just a pause on the future they had envisioned and planned together. The parent of a child with severe brain damage told me she cannot let go of the hope that one day there will be a cure, perhaps a brain transplant, that will allow her to have her "real" son back. Now I am not suggesting we should lose all hope for the future, but the point I am trying to make is that there is a time when we need to grieve what we wanted the relationship to be and accept what it actually is. By hanging on so tightly to the past, or to how we want the future to be, we are not allowing ourselves to appreciate and accept life in the present moment, and we can't redefine the relationship in a way that is sustaining and mutually fulfilling.

PRACTICAL EXERCISE — REFLECT ON YOUR LIFE

Take the time to reflect on where you've been in your life and where you are at now. In your journal, write your autobiography. In other words, write out the story of your life up until today. It will be easier if you write the story of your life in increments of five years, starting at birth. Once you are done, look at the five-year period prior to when your caregiving role began and reflect on how the relationship with your care recipient has changed, for the better and for the worse.

REFLECTIVE QUESTIONS

- Who are you as a person (beyond your caregiving role)?
- How have your life events shaped you as a caregiver?
- How has your caregiving experience changed you as an individual, and how has it changed the relationship with your care recipient?

THE NEW NORMAL

The change in relationship dynamics can bring out both the good and the bad in us. It can challenge us in the worst ways as well as in the greatest ways. When experiencing a relationship that is going from what we want it to be to something entirely different, caregivers can feel a wide range of emotions. They may feel stuck, disappointed, resentful, and even become depressed, as discussed in the previous chapter. There is a grieving process that happens when you lose the ideals of the past and the illusion of the future you had envisioned. Some are able to grieve the old relationship — the one they expected and wanted — and create a new relationship that is different but still fulfilling. Others cannot. Either way, whatever your normal life was, it no longer is, as you can see from the stories below:

> "When my daughter was born with autism, my life changed in ways I could not have imagined. I could no longer work, and with one income, we could no longer sustain our lifestyle. My husband and I started fighting about money, about how things should be done, and about almost everything. We couldn't seem to handle the pressures of constant caregiving. It took its toll, and we were not able to find a new way of being together under these extreme conditions. My family has fallen apart. We are in the process of getting a divorce. My life is in shambles, and I don't see how I will be able to move forward from this."

> "We'd been married almost fifteen years when my wife developed a serious mental illness. In many ways I've lost the woman I married, but somehow, we're muddling our way through it. We've created a new kind of relationship where we don't look back at what we had, or think about how things were supposed to be, but instead try to find the blessings in the life we are actually living right now. We have found a way to accept the situation and to create a new vision for our future together."

> "My husband and I both grieve our own ideas of what our lives should have been in different ways. I am not sure either one of us has come to acceptance yet. In some ways I'm in denial and still believe that this is just a phase, and that we will be back on

track soon. It's hard to accept that this is my new normal. I am still grieving, and I'm not sure this grief will pass. Letting go of my old visions and dreams is terribly difficult, but I hope someday I can let go of the anger, sadness, fear, guilt, and sense of failure. Perhaps someday I will embrace this new path and actually get excited about the unknown destination we are headed toward. But for now, I grieve."

You may need to take some time to mourn the loss of the relationship you had, as well as the hopes and dreams you held. If you can no longer have the experiences you'd planned, it is important to deal with the sense of loss so it doesn't prevent you from creating new hopes and dreams. When letting go of expectations of how life was supposed to be, people can often find new ways to live out some of their old dreams as well as create new ones. Perhaps your care recipient does not have much time left, and the best possible future is to experience love and compassion in their final days. Or if they are deteriorating rapidly, perhaps it is to receive good care and be surrounded by positive energy for the duration of their illness. And in other cases, it is a matter of grieving what was and looking at how you can create a brighter future as individuals and in the caregiving relationship.

PRACTICAL EXERCISE — CREATE A NEW VISION

Take some time to journal about how you thought your future would be and how your caregiving role has caused this vision to change. Once you are done, journal about any new hopes and dreams you might have.

REFLECTIVE QUESTIONS

- How can you create a compelling and sustainable future in light of your caregiving role?
- How would your ideal "new normal" look given your caregiving situation?
- Are there specific action steps you can take to work toward making your new dreams a reality?

INTIMACY

We tend to think of intimacy in a sexual sense, but intimacy refers to the level of closeness and connection we have in any relationship. Obviously, in a sexual relationship, there is an added component, but between partners there are many other components as well, including the mental, emotional, physical, and spiritual connection. Within families, there are these same areas of intimacy, and when caregiving roles alter the level of intimacy in a relationship, problems inevitably arise. When a loved one's disability deprives you of the intimacy you once enjoyed, or had expected to share in the future, the relationship can be completely transformed, leaving you feeling unhappy and unfulfilled, as in this woman's case:

> "In many ways, I feel widowed. Intimacy and partnership with my husband has been lost since the onset of his dementia. Even in our conversations, he has lost the ability to pick up nuances and the wordplay that was a big part of our mental and emotional connection. We have no more sexual connection either, but it's not really about that. I just don't feel much connection with him on any level."

In some instances, a loved one's disability can actually create a level of connection that is above and beyond what existed before. Here are a few examples to illustrate:

> "When my husband confided that he was suffering from PTSD, it was a relief in some ways. He finally opened up to me. I still remember the night he told me what was really going on with him. It was an immediate realization that all of our struggles, the reason we were falling away from each other, had nothing to do with me, with him not loving me, or with him having an affair or wanting to end the marriage. This thing that was tearing us apart finally had a name. I could understand it. I could work with it. In tears, we held each other closer than we had in years. I told him I would be there for him and that we'd get through it together. His illness, as difficult and disabling as it is, has brought us to a whole new level of intimacy. He finally let me in. He let me care for him. I could be part of his

life again. Now we talk. I listen on a deeper level. I have learned to support him emotionally."

"When my son got into a car accident, he went from physically and emotionally distant to needing my help. I got to be a mom again. We reconnected in ways I never thought we would. He talked to me. He needed me. It was almost a year before he could walk again, and two years before he regained his independence. But even now, he still asks for my help with things. He comes around. A whole new bond has been created. So for me, becoming his caregiver was a blessing in disguise. I went from thinking I was losing my son to realizing that I was actually getting him back."

"When my father had a stroke, I got to see a side of him I never knew existed. Suddenly, we found ourselves spending a lot of time together. We had to overcome awkward situations, but as he regained his speech, he told me stories about his life that I'd never heard before. He became a real person to me versus the mysterious man that I'd lived with my whole life and yet knew virtually nothing about."

"My mother's illness has allowed me to be more open about my fears, my struggles, and to talk more openly with her than ever before. After all these years, we are building a deeper level of trust that neither of us had ever experienced before."

"My diagnosis actually brought us closer together. Our life before I found out I had Parkinson's was falling apart. We were together as a couple yet living separate lives. We were drifting further and further apart. We had not slept in the same bed for years. Any of his attempts to come together were met with resistance and anger from me. After my diagnosis, we began to try to repair our relationship. We spent more time together, we made family a priority, and we tried to understand each other more. I need him, and he needs to be needed. He wants to support me. He reassures me he is in it for the long haul — for better or for worse — and that we would get through anything together. And we are. With some hiccups along the way. I just wish we could have had this level of intimacy without this awful disease, but I guess we needed something drastic to find our way back to each other."

The fact is, human beings need and want intimacy. We thrive on connection, and when intimacy is lacking, we feel unfulfilled. Caregiving fundamentally alters the level of intimacy in any type of relationship, sometimes for the better and other times for the worse. As you can see from the examples above, the start of a caregiving relationship does not need to signal the end of intimacy. Consider the possibility of redefining intimacy and creating a new type of connection in your relationship.

PRACTICAL EXERCISE — CREATE MORE CONNECTION

Separate a sheet of paper into two columns. In one column, make a list of all of the things *you* are currently saying, thinking, and doing that are disconnecting you from your care recipient. In the other column, make a list of all of the things you are currently saying, thinking, and doing that strengthen the connection with your care recipient. Throughout the day, give some serious consideration to what you are bringing to the relationship, and commit to doing more things from your connection list and less from your disconnection list. Remember, it is your choice whether you choose connection or disconnection, and that choice will significantly impact how you feel about your care recipient. Before going to bed, write about at least one instance where you chose to create connection and one instance where you chose to create disconnection.

REFLECTIVE QUESTIONS

In all of your thoughts, words, and actions today, ask yourself:

- Is this serving to create connection or disconnection in my caregiving relationship?
- Why do I choose to create disconnection?
- What is contributing to my choice to connect and/or disconnect?

SEXUAL INTIMACY

Although intimacy does not always involve sex, I do want to briefly touch on the impact caregiving can have on sexual intimacy. Some couples lose sexual intimacy because one partner is sick, disabled, or otherwise no longer able to engage in a sexual relationship. In other situations where both partners are healthy, the caregiver is just too tired to share any kind of sexual intimacy after taking care of someone else all day long, along with taking care of their regular responsibilities. There is no time or energy left over to sit and talk, to relax together, go for walks, enjoy each other's company, much less have sex. Regardless of the specific situation, sexual intimacy is a complex issue that can be very difficult to navigate. As you can see from the statements below, for couples who are in a caregiving situation, the issues around sexual intimacy are quite varied and real:

"I can't really complain about my lack of sex when my husband is bedridden and in constant pain. Sex is the least of his worries, and I understand it should be the least of mine, but the reality is that I still have sexual needs that he can't meet."

"This is going to sound really selfish, but when my wife got sick, I hated that I was the one suddenly making all the dinners, doing the laundry, cleaning, driving the kids everywhere, helping with homework, and everything else that comes with running a household. I was the husband and the wife, the mom and the dad. I was meeting everyone's needs, but no one was meeting mine any more. How can I even think about my needs when I can still live a normal life? And if I dare mention sex, I'd surely be considered a heartless bastard."

"I don't have the time, energy, or interest in sex. I don't even know this side of myself any more. It's like my sexuality has gone dormant."

"My husband is in the early to mid stages of Alzheimer's disease. He still wants to have a sexual relationship, but I don't see him in that light anymore. I feel more like his mother or his nurse, but not like his wife. This situation is very difficult because I still have sexual needs, and so does he, but I just don't feel it with *him* any more."

"Sex has become a constant battle. My husband wants sex, and I don't. After taking care of my disabled child *and* my sick mother all day, believe me, sex is the last thing on my mind when I crawl into bed at night. This is an extreme source of frustration for both of us. Part of me worries he will look for sex elsewhere, and yet another part of me doesn't care."

PRACTICAL EXERCISE — REDEFINE INTIMACY

Start by writing out what intimacy means to you in the context of your care-giving relationship. In other words, if you had the ideal level of connection with your care recipient given the circumstances, what would that look like on all levels — mentally, emotionally, physically, socially, spiritually, etc.? If you are also in a romantic relationship, complete this exercise in the context of that relationship, adding the area of sexual intimacy.

REFLECTIVE QUESTIONS

- How would you know if you had a good level of intimacy, closeness, and connection with your care recipient and/or partner?

- How can you foster intimacy and connection with your care recipient and/or partner? What new activities and experiences could you find to bond over?

- How can you meet your needs for intimacy in healthy ways, either within your caregiving relationship or through other productive means?

VALUES AND NEEDS FULFILLMENT

As much as some caregiving experiences result in increased intimacy, many do not. Often, our sick or disabled loved one loses the ability to meet our needs. To make matters worse, while caregiving, we often end up putting our own needs on the back burner as we put all of our time and energy into meeting someone else's needs.

When we have unmet needs, sexual, emotional, or otherwise, we start seeking ways to meet those needs. Some turn to other family and friends to fulfill their needs. Others find unhealthy solutions to meet their needs. In fact, the solutions we come up with can serve to exacerbate our feelings of disconnection and breed further disconnection, such that we are further away from each other on all levels.

PRACTICAL EXERCISE — DEFINE YOUR NEEDS AND VALUES

Separate a sheet of paper in two columns. List all of your needs in one column and all of your values in the other. List as many as you can in no particular order. Keep going until you can't think of anything more. Don't read any further until you've completed your lists. Once you've thoroughly completed your lists, put your needs in order of importance as quickly as you can without giving it too much thought. Then do the same thing with your values list.

REFLECTIVE QUESTIONS

When looking at your needs and values lists, take the top six from each list and ask yourself:

- Are your most important needs currently being fulfilled through your relationships and experiences? If not, look at the needs that are not being met and think of ways to meet those needs in a healthy way.

- Are you living in accordance to your values? If not, with which values are you out of alignment? How can you get back into alignment with these important values?

- How are you taking responsibility for meeting your own needs and ensuring that you are being true to your values?

If you are in a romantic relationship, it can be very beneficial to have your partner complete these exercises as well. Then compare notes and see how your needs and values line up. This can form a very good foundation for negotiating how to meet each other's most important needs or to brainstorm other ways to honour each other's needs and values.

PROMOTE BALANCE AND INDEPENDENCE

Over time, relationships develop a certain balance and equilibrium. There is a sense of predictability that creates a feeling of peace and harmony. However, when illness strikes, the balance of the relationship is often shattered. In some caregiving instances, the care recipient becomes completely dependent and can no longer carry any of the responsibilities that they used to or meet the needs as typically expected in this type of relationship. In other cases, the care recipient can still maintain some of the responsibilities and meet the needs of the relationship, fully or partially, or take new ones on. With that said, sometimes the caregiver does not allow them to. They can overprotect and take away more roles and responsibilities from the care recipient than is necessary, thus rendering them almost invalid. This negatively affects all aspects of the relationship.

While it may be true that you can do things more efficiently than your care recipient, it is important to recognize what they are still able to do and to allow them to contribute to the relationship in whatever ways they can. No one can thrive without meaning and purpose. No one can maintain optimism without hopes and dreams. No one will feel fulfilled without some sense of control over their environment. So give your care recipient as much power and independence as possible, given their unique situation. If they are completely disabled, perhaps you can still give them simple choices or get their assistance with things they can still manage. For example, with supervision, my grandmother could still assist with the care of my children. It gave her great joy to change a diaper — a task I was more than happy to give away. She also enjoyed helping with food preparation, and even though I could chop the vegetables at twice the speed, it saved me time because I could do other things while she took care of the veggies. I could see that she appreciated being trusted with a task, especially an important one, such as one that involved the children. It made her feel needed. Everyone needs to feel worthy, wanted, and needed. When someone loses their sense of identity, their sense of purpose and their value in the relationship, they start to buy into their role as a sick person, because it's all that's left. They may well be ill, but that is not all of who they are. Therefore, it is very important to ensure you are promoting as much balance and independence as possible.

Resist the urge to do too much for your care recipient. Allow them to gain as much freedom and independence as possible, given the unique set of circumstances.

PRACTICAL EXERCISE — CREATE MORE BALANCE AND INDEPENDENCE

Before you can create more balance in the caregiving relationship and return some independence to your care recipient, it is important to first look at what you are getting out of doing too much. In your journal, make a thorough list of the reasons you've created dependency in certain areas of your caregiving relationship (e.g., the need to be needed, etc.)

REFLECTIVE QUESTIONS

- What choices and decisions could you put back into the hands of your care recipient?
- What tasks could your care recipient be doing or helping with?
- In what other ways can you promote balance and independence in your caregiving relationship?

THE DANCE OF GIVING AND RECEIVING

Obviously, in order to give, someone has to receive. Giving and receiving is a continuous cycle with giving as the outflow and receiving as the inflow. We often talk about the gift of giving, but how often do we hear anything about the gift of receiving? For some reason, we love to give and yet find receiving to be quite uncomfortable. How many of us give gracefully but receive awkwardly? Why is that? Why do we block the inflow of energy instead of accepting it wholeheartedly? I also wonder what we are taking away from the giver when we do not openly receive. For example, if the giver is excited to authentically give to you out of appreciation and love, what happens when you block it?

The caregiver role can often feel like an all-giving, no-receiving type of situation where the caregiver gives, gives, gives, and the care recipient takes, takes, takes. This may be inevitable in certain types of caregiving situations, such as those where the care recipient truly is unable to contribute to the relationship. But if this is the case, it is important for the caregiver to be in receiving mode in other relationships, as well as to give to themselves in whatever ways possible. The channel of giving and receiving must be open on both ends, or negative thoughts, emotions, and energy will start to erode the relationship between the caregiver and care recipient and can also permeate other relationships.

PRACTICAL EXERCISE — PRACTICE RECEIVING

As a caregiver, chances are you do not need more practice in the giving department. However, there is a good chance you could use some practice receiving. Therefore, this is your challenge ... if at all possible, get away from caregiving for at least three days and treat yourself to a retreat of some sort. One where you have plenty of time to sit back, relax, think about yourself, receive some special treatment. This does not have to be an expensive retreat. I once took a retreat in my friend's spare bedroom, where I spent four days completely alone with just a journal and a pen (more on this in Chapter Six).

REFLECTIVE QUESTIONS

- Beyond typical self-care activities (e.g., bath, massage, meditation), how can you create opportunities to practice gracefully receiving from others?

- In what ways or areas of your life do you find it most difficult to receive from others?

- In what other ways can you give and receive from yourself?

CONCLUSION

Sometimes a big part of rebuilding a relationship is the ability to let go of previously defined roles and responsibilities. It's about allowing ourselves to grieve what was and what might have been. It's being able to let someone care for us without feeling like we always need to be the strong one or the one in control. Giving other people the opportunity to take on the caregiver role along with us and allowing them to feel needed can create a more positive flow of energy in the relationship. Perhaps there are still ways your care recipient can contribute to the relationship and offer value to you. Perhaps you can receive from each other in certain ways. We all have our own unique needs and values, and we must honour them. Once we do, we can build a new relationship with ourselves and with each other — one that is fulfilling and can take the relationship to a different level, to a "new normal." There will still be challenges, however; where once you were battling against the tides, you may now find yourself riding them out together.

CHAPTER FOUR

CAREGIVER COMMUNICATION

"Most people do not listen
with the intent to understand;
they listen with the intent to reply."

—Stephen R. Covey

Effective communication is a key way to strengthening your relationships. It is through communication that we establish and maintain them. It is how we share our thoughts, feelings, hopes, dreams, fears, etc. Being able to effectively communicate your experiences and how you are being affected, both positively and negatively, can allow you to enjoy more of the rewards and benefits of your caregiving relationship and serve to create more fulfilment in all areas of your life.

Most of us think of communication as talking, which is partly true, but listening is where the magic happens. Of course, someone has to be talking in order for the other to be listening, but keep in mind, when you are the listener, not only do you need to listen to what is being said, but also to what is not being said. As you've undoubtedly learned, a large percentage of our communication is nonverbal. With this in mind, as a caregiver you must listen not only with your ears, but also with your eyes and your intuition. When caring for a real, living, breathing human being, give them your true, focused, undivided attention — your full concentration, consideration, and alertness — when communicating. Every conversation is an opportunity to heal, learn, and grow.

The tips in this chapter are aimed at giving you strategies on how to communicate with your care recipient so you can provide the best possible care for them and avoid the miscommunications that result in frustration for both of you. It is also intended to help you share your thoughts and feelings in ways that allow you to clear out negative emotions and effectively communicate your needs.

In my own caregiving situation, my grandmother could no longer engage in higher-level conversations. Over time, her conversational skills were whittled down to the same five stories and three or four repetitive questions. This may also be the case for you, but even if your care recipient can no longer communicate, these strategies will help you communicate more productively in all of your relationships.

SEEK TO UNDERSTAND

As a caregiver, seeking to understand what your care recipient is actually trying to say will spare you time and energy, as well as the frustrations so many of us experience from miscommunication and/or lack of communication. As with the quote at the beginning of this chapter, many people are not really listening but instead are waiting to talk. They are not hearing or seeking to understand the other person's perspective but are anxiously waiting to give their own opinions. This approach usually leaves both parties to the conversation feeling as though they were not heard, understood, or acknowledged. It often causes us to get defensive, repeat our point of view more forcefully, or shut down and stop talking altogether. When we are going around and around the same topic, repeating ourselves and never getting anywhere, we must ask ourselves if we are really listening and truly hearing what the other person is saying. Perhaps they are not listening either, but one thing I can almost guarantee is once a person feels heard, they will likely be more open and receptive to what you have to say. Allow them time to explain their point of view without interrupting or defending yourself. Give the benefit of the doubt and stand in the possibility of being wrong, so you can at least hear their side of the "story." Here is a quick example to illustrate how jumping straight into your own side of the story without seeking to understand can lead to trouble and how a simple shift in approach can lead to better understanding and ultimately to better solutions:

SCENARIO 1

Caregiver (CG): You need to take a bath and change your clothes every day. If you don't, I'm not taking you out in public any more.

Care Recipient (CR): I'm tired of you telling me what to do. You're not the boss!

SCENARIO 2

CG: Mom, you and I seem to have a different opinion on how often you should bathe and change your clothes. I'm wondering if you could tell me how you see things.

CR: I slipped the other day when I was getting out of the shower and almost fell. I'm afraid I will hurt myself and become even more dependent on you. Plus, every time I change my clothes, it makes more laundry for you, and you always say how you hate doing laundry.

CG: I didn't know you'd almost slipped, or that you felt this way. I'm wondering if we could talk more about this, and I'd also like to share with you my concerns so we can try to come up with solutions together.

PRACTICE EXERCISE — LISTEN AND ASK

Do as little speaking as possible today. When you do speak, use open-ended questions with the goal of clarifying and steering the conversation to a deeper level. See if you can remain in a genuine state of curiosity. Instead of defending or explaining your own points, ask questions like:

- What's it like for you when...?
- Can you tell me more?
- Can you share your thoughts on...?
- What else are you experiencing?
- What are you worried might happen if...?

REFLECTIVE QUESTIONS

- Do you listen to understand, or are you simply waiting to speak?
- Do you interrupt, change the subject, or multitask while someone is speaking to you?
- Do you pay attention to shifts in facial expressions and body language when someone is talking to you?

CREATE OPENINGS FOR REAL CONVERSATION

Create openings in the conversation to talk about what is really going on. You may ask how they are doing, and they may say "fine." Then you can say, "How are you *really* doing?" That way they know you really want to hear the answer. Once they answer, ask if there is anything else, ask a follow-up question, or rephrase your question to something more specific. For example: "On a scale of 1 to 5, 1 being the worst you've been since your illness began and 5 being the best, how would you rate how you are feeling today?" Then listen carefully to their response and check for understanding. As a therapist, I am trained in techniques like restating and paraphrasing. Restating is quite simple. It's just a matter of repeating exactly what the person said, then checking if they have anything to add or correct. For example, if you say, "You seem agitated. What's going on?" and the person answers, "You are not listening to me," then you might answer, "When you say I am not listening to you, what exactly do you mean? Can you give an example?"

Paraphrasing is slightly different. It is trying to capture what the person said without repeating what they said word for word, and then checking again for understanding. In the previous example, paraphrasing may sound something like, "I am hearing that you feel like I'm not getting what you're trying to say. Is that right?" Here's another quick example. If you say, "How are you?" and the person answers, "I'm fine, but busy." You might answer, "When you say you're fine, but busy ... what exactly does that mean for you?" Or in the case of paraphrasing, you might say, "Sounds like you're busy but doing okay. Am I getting that right?"

If you sense the other person is not being honest in their response, you may probe a bit further. For example, if they say they are fine but clearly do not look fine, you might say, "When you say you're fine, I sense there might be something more going on. Is there anything you'd like to talk about?" Or you might say, "You don't really seem fine. Is something bothering you?"

If they continue to be reluctant to open up, back off but let them know you are available to talk and help, if and when they are ready. Let it go for the time being. Perhaps you can circle back to it later if an opportunity arises.

These techniques show your care recipient you are hearing and seeking to understand what they are saying, as well as respectfully trying to uncover any thoughts or feelings they might not be expressing. All too often, we make assumptions about what we think we are hearing and do not bother to clarify. This can easily lead to further misunderstandings and breakdowns in communication. By looking someone in the eye and digging deeper with open-ended questions, you are providing opportunity for clarification. It is also creating an opportunity for your care recipient to expand their thoughts and feelings, which also helps them express things they have not yet had a chance to acknowledge or talk about.

Regardless of how developed your communication skills may be, the most important thing to remember is to be authentic and genuinely want to know what's going on. This means going beyond the superficial and creating opportunities to talk about what really matters. What is the person feeling, fearing, and carrying? Actively listening in such a deep way shows you are committed to trying to understand their needs, values, and interests.

Many people avoid real conversations because they believe it may lead to hurt feelings, judgements, or conflict. They may feel the need to protect the person and the relationship. However, a healthy relationship is being able to have honest conversations that matter, where both parties can listen with compassion and freely express their thoughts and feelings without blame. This doesn't mean you'll always like what you hear or that you'll agree on everything, but there is a much better chance of working together toward a satisfying compromise through real conversations.

When creating an opening for real conversation, make sure to do it face-to-face — *not* by text or by email. If you cannot have the conversation in person, then do it face-to-face using technology (Skype, FaceTime, Zoom, etc.). Approach the conversation with a welcoming, open tone and not from a place of aggression, defensiveness, or passivity. You might even start by saying, "I need to have an honest conversation with you." This gives the person the opportunity to realize this is not going to be a run-of-the-mill conversation. You can also ask, "Is this a good time?" This question allows the person to determine whether or not they are ready for the talk, showing them their time and energy is a priority for you. Recognizing mutual convenience and waiting for a good time to have a real conversation can be the difference between a positive outcome and a negative one.

PRACTICAL EXERCISE — CREATE AN OPENING FOR REAL CONVERSATION

If there is a conversation that has been spinning around in your mind, go out and have it today. Once you open the conversation, ask to be fully heard and let the person know that you want to fully hear them out as well. Acknowledge the reason you want to have this conversation is because the person matters to you, and you want to get their perspective because you might be missing important pieces of information. Then let them know what's on your mind without faulting or making them wrong. Once you've expressed yourself and let them know how you've been affected by this situation, ask how they see things and genuinely listen to what they have to say. Their first reaction may be defensive or dismissive, but if you can persevere and persuade them to keep talking, you will get to the deeper layers of the issues from their perspective. You can respect and strengthen the relationship, even if you have differing points of view, by asking questions such as:

- What parts of this situation do we see in common?
- Why do you think we see things differently?
- Do you feel there is anything I might be missing or misunderstanding?

REFLECTIVE QUESTIONS

- Do you avoid real conversations? If so, why?
- What assumptions do you have about having real conversations?
- What do you fear will happen if you start having real conversations?

IDENTIFY THE UNDERLYING EMOTIONS

Another great communication strategy is to mention an emotion you are seeing or sensing. For example, "You look like you're feeling sad today." The person may say, "I am sad," and explain why. Or they may explain that they are tired, or perhaps feeling another emotion. Regardless of the response, identifying the underlying emotion you are sensing creates a space for a conversation about emotions by letting the person know you are noticing how they are feeling and interested in hearing more about it. It is almost certain that there is an internal conversation going on in your loved one's mind, and this conversation has nowhere to go except around and around in their head. You can help them get this conversation out in the open so they can process it on a deeper level and feel supported in whatever they are feeling and fearing. All it requires is genuine curiosity and authenticity tied in with good questions and great listening.

Sample Conversation:

Caregiver (CG): You look angry today.

Care Recipient (CR): It's not that. I'm just in pain. My back is really sore, and I can barely sit up. (Flinches as he touches his back)

CG: Wow, sounds painful and frustrating.

CR: It is very frustrating to be in constant pain. I can't sleep, can't do the things I want to do, plus I worry about never getting back to normal.

CG: What else do you worry about?

CR: I'm afraid I will become dependent on everyone and be a burden. I feel lonely even when people are around. I feel angry that I am the one who is sick while everyone gets to continue on with their lives.

CG: That's a lot to process. It's hard to put myself in your shoes, because I haven't been in your situation, but I think I would be lonely and resentful too if I saw everyone going about their business while I'm lying in a hospital bed in pain and unable to do the things I normally do. I'm thinking it would feel like life is going on without me.

CR: That's exactly how it feels! And then mix in the fear of never getting your health back and throw major pain into it, which makes me feel like a big complainer.

CG: I guess it would be hard to focus on the positive when pain just keeps reminding you of where you're at. Is there anything I can do to help? What's really frustrating for me is not knowing what to do or not do.

CR: Well, just letting me talk about what's really going on is helpful. I hate it when people come by to talk about the weather, pretending like everything is fine when we all know it's not.

CG: Sometimes I don't know what to say, and it seems safer to keep to the superficial stuff. I never know if you want to talk or if talking about it makes things worse.

CR: Talking about what's going on definitely helps.

CG: Talking just doesn't seem to be enough. I want to do something more. You know what I mean?

CR: Yeah but trust me, it is enough. Soon I'm going to be getting back on my feet, and I promise I will let you know what I need.

CG: You said you're having a hard time sitting up. Did you need some help getting something or getting into a more comfortable position?

CR: You could hand me that cup if you don't mind, but truthfully, I just can't find a good comfortable position right now.

Feelings need an outlet. They don't necessarily need fixing. Once the underlying feelings are fully acknowledged, it's as if they are free to go and can sometimes vanish back to wherever they came from. Other times, the emotions will stick around, but at least the person knows there is someone willing to listen and help them process what they are experiencing. In other words, they have an outlet. Asking about your care recipient's emotions lets them know you care and that they are not alone.

PRACTICAL EXERCISE — CALL OUT EMOTIONS

Talking about feelings is scary for many people and can be quite uncomfortable. They may not trust themselves to know what to do if things get emotional or heated. Perhaps you consider it weak or even a waste of time to talk about emotions. If this is you, start in a low-risk way by calling out emotions you are more comfortable with. Perhaps pain, anxiety, or confusion would be more comfortable emotions to start with. Regardless of which emotions you choose, your task today is to call out as many emotions as possible. If you're having a conversation and notice a shift in emotions, identify the emotion you think you're seeing or sensing and ask about it.

REFLECTIVE QUESTIONS

- Do you trust yourself to handle other people's emotions? Do you trust yourself to handle your own emotions?
- What risks do you believe are involved in sharing emotions?
- What benefits do you believe are associated with sharing emotions?

DON'T BE QUICK TO OFFER SOLUTIONS

Caregivers are often master problem-solvers and often feel rewarded by effectively managing a situation and making it better. Many of us in the above scenario between caregiver and care recipient would go straight to trying to adjust the person's position and helping them get more comfortable in bed. There's nothing wrong with that, but it is also important to take the time to truly hear and understand what's really going on and not jump straight in to offering solutions. Ultimately, a solution may be needed, but skipping the acknowledgement and understanding part of the process is a huge mistake. As in the example conversation above, when the care recipient said his back was sore and he could barely sit up, it might make you feel better to try to adjust pillows or to do something more concrete to solve the problem. However, as you can see, it would bypass the deeper emotional needs. In many cases, the person may simply need to know you care, that they are important to you, and that their feelings matter. They may simply need to be heard and have someone acknowledge what they are going through. At the end of the conversation, you can still offer solutions, as long as you're truly hearing the problem at its deeper level. Often, the problem is not what is being said at the surface level; it's what's under that first or second layer. Don't be afraid to dig in, ask more questions, check your understanding, and show that you have heard what they are saying and are making an honest effort to understand.

Sometimes we become frustrated because we can't fix a problem, and the person keeps repeating the same problem over and over, but I can almost guarantee if they are repeating themselves it's because they feel you are not getting it. So step out of problem-solving mode for a while and just listen. This will take pressure off you and allow you to learn more about what is really going on. You will likely leave the conversation with a much better understanding of what is affecting your care recipient, why they are acting the way they are, and also how to support them better.

PRACTICAL EXERCISE — HAVE A CONVERSATION WITHOUT OFFERING ANY SOLUTIONS

Have a conversation with your care recipient without offering any solutions whatsoever. Regardless of the person's words or actions, meet them with compassion, dignity, and respect. Try to read them and ask questions that will help drive the conversation to a deeper level. Listen attentively without interruptions. Make them feel heard and understood without offering solutions. When asking questions, allow the person time to reflect and to formulate a response. Be patient and let them communicate their difficulties, their challenges, and their emotions. Don't assume or ask another question until you've given them time and space to fully express and communicate what they really need to say. Understand the person needs to be heard and might also need time to organize thoughts internally before expressing them outwardly, especially when fears and emotions are running high. Allow plenty of space for silence, and when you feel like saying something, pause for a moment. Count to ten in your mind to give them that extra window of opportunity for them to add to what they were saying. Show genuine interest in their thoughts, feelings, and concerns. Instead of fixing, just listen.

REFLECTIVE QUESTIONS

Once your care recipient has fully expressed themselves, try to help them come up with their own solutions. Even if you think you have the perfect solution, see if you can get them to find their own by asking questions like:

- Have you ever been in this situation before? If so, what did you do? If not, do you know anyone who has? If so, what did they do?
- What have you tried so far?
- Do you have ideas on what you could do to make things better?

GET REAL AND SHOW VULNERABILITY

This can be tricky, depending what your loved one is going through, and we often hesitate to share our own feelings. Perhaps you feel you have to be strong at all times and be the rock, but if you won't talk about how you're really feeling, your loved one may not feel safe in doing so either. As a mental health client told me, "If you don't talk to me about your fears, I probably won't feel safe talking to you about mine."

So let your care recipient in on some of your struggles and allow them to provide you with some emotional support as well. In the example conversation above, when the care recipient says he is frustrated about people going on with their lives, you may say something like:

> CG: I'm surprised to hear you say that, because I always thought when someone is very sick, the best thing to do is act normal and stay upbeat. You know, keep it light since the person already has enough to deal with.

> CR: For me, that's probably the worst thing you can do.

> CG: Wow, I didn't know that. I figured you had enough to deal with without hearing about how worried I am about you.

> CR: When people act like nothing is going on, it makes me feel like they don't care.

> CG: The truth is I seriously don't know what I'll do if you don't heal from this, and I'm scared.

> CR: I'm scared too. Soooooo scared.

> CG: Help me understand what it's like from your perspective.

Now, this conversation might be fraught with tears, but getting it out in the open is just that, so you can talk about what's already going on inside you (and inside the other person). Otherwise, these internal conversations have nowhere to go. They just spin around and around. There may not be a solution to the fears one or both of you are feeling, but this is creating an opening for those emotions to get out into the open authentically.

Try to access feelings of vulnerability that the care recipient might be feeling by projecting honesty and authenticity. This allows the care recipient to be open and trust you to support them through this difficult and scary time. To do this, share your own fears and insecurities and ask about theirs. Don't try to pull a "fast one" or avoid difficult questions or conversations. Be open and honest in delivering the bad news along with the good, using tact, discretion, and compassion. And don't make promises you can't keep. As a side note, if you are caregiving on a professional level, you will need to be very careful with self-disclosure. My rule of thumb is, sharing your current struggles is an absolute no-no — do not put your problems on your client/patient and look to them for support. However, if you have a relatable past experience that you have successfully resolved, it may be appropriate to share parts of your story in an effort to build trust, offer hope, and connect on a deeper level. As a professional, self-disclosure should only be used in an effort to meet the client/patient's needs and improve their mental and emotional state, not to meet your own needs.

REFLECTIVE QUESTIONS

- What has stopped you in the past from being authentic?
- What has stopped you in the past from being vulnerable?
- What fears do you have around hearing someone's real fears and concerns?

ENCOURAGE TEARS

Don't stop the conversation when the tears start. You may worry that if the person has a meltdown, they won't be able to get themselves back together again. But I can assure you after having many people bawl on my shoulder, snot on my shirt, and use every last tissue in my Kleenex box, I have never had one person not recover from it. There is already a storm of emotions inside them. You are not creating the storm by asking the tough questions. You are not "making" them cry. You are simply holding the space for the storm to come out. If it continues to brew without an outlet, it cannot pass. It stays trapped. When a person starts to cry, refrain from attempts to shift them into positive thinking or into platitudes about how this too shall pass or making jokes and trying to get them in a better mood. Instead, you can say things like, "You are safe," "I'm here," "Let the tears come." Give them the honour of being fully present in their time of need and keep passing the tissue and offering a hug or a shoulder to cry on until the storm passes. I promise if you can stand in the middle of someone else's storm and be the beacon of light guiding them back to safety, it will be highly rewarding for you and extremely healing for them. You will likely feel relieved at not holding the responsibility of fixing them and relieved at knowing that it's okay for us all to fall apart at times. This is not to say we shouldn't try to offer positive messages, but when the tears start to flow, see if you can get comfortable with allowing them and even encouraging them. Remember, you don't have to fix anything — just hold the space.

You may not always feel able to talk about your emotions or to hear about someone else's, but make sure to tell them why. You may say, "This is important to me, but right now I'm not able to talk about it because I'm _____(fill in the blank)."

PRACTICE EXERCISE — BRING ON THE TEARS

The next time you are in a conversation and notice someone getting tearful, ask genuinely about what is making them tearful. If they cry harder, let them know that it's okay to keep the tears coming. Ask them what those tears are saying.

REFLECTIVE QUESTIONS

- How comfortable are you with crying in front of other people?
- How comfortable are you with other people's tears?
- How did it feel to let someone cry without trying to cheer them up or fix the problem?

PAY ATTENTION TO YOUR INTENTIONS

Sometimes we say things or ask questions with hidden intentions. For example, you may ask your diabetic mother something like, "Mom, did you eat this candy?" as you're holding the candy wrapper in your hand, knowing full well she ate it. Instead of asking a question you already know the answer to and generating feelings of shame or defensiveness, here's another approach you could try. It's called the OPEN communication strategy:

> O stands for Observation
>
> P stands for Perception
>
> E stands for Emotion
>
> N stands for Need

CG: When you eat candies (observation), I think you're going to get sick (perception), and I get scared (emotion) because I still need and want my mom around (need).

CR: I'm trying, I really am, but I have cravings, and I just can't control them sometimes.

CG: Tell me more about that. I really want to understand, because when I see you eating things you're not supposed to eat (observation), I think you're trying to hurt yourself (perception), and I feel like you're abandoning me (emotion), and I need to try to understand where you're coming from and what's really going on for you (need).

CR: I'm not trying to hurt you or myself, it's just hard because I'm alone and bored and there are things I'm not supposed to eat all around me.

CG: Is there anything we can do to make this easier for you?

PRACTICAL EXERCISE — SET AN INTENTION

Before having the next conversation with your care recipient, sit down and think with a very clear focus about what your intention for the conversation is. Write it down and honestly look at your intention. If your intention is to heal, connect, and bring understanding to the issue at hand, you're ready. If it's to manipulate, to get your own way, or to try to make them understand your point of view, then perhaps consider waiting to have the conversation *or* consider calling yourself out on your intentions. For example, as you begin the sample conversation above, you might say something like, "I want to talk to you about something but realize I'm coming at this the wrong way. I want you to see things my way, but I know this probably won't help us find a solution that works for both of us. I'm telling you this because I might need help having this conversation in a way that works for you too." When you open the conversation with an up-front admission of your intentions, the other person is likely to let their guard down somewhat because you're being honest and asking for help.

REFLECTIVE QUESTIONS

- What topics do you have most trouble communicating about with your care recipient?

- Do you try to get your point across using hidden intentions or underhanded methods?

- In what ways do you try to manipulate your care recipient instead of having a direct conversation?

CONCLUSION

It can be difficult to know what and what not to say in certain caregiving situations. We often feel like we are walking on eggshells. We don't want to upset our loved one. We might not want to confront them. We want to avoid burdening them with our thoughts and feelings. Although it can be difficult to broach a touchy subject and engage in what might be a difficult conversation, learning to communicate from a sincere, honest place is incredibly empowering and healing for both the care recipient and the caregiver. If your care recipient does not have the cognitive capacity to engage in these types of conversations, find someone you can talk to about your deeper thoughts and feelings, perhaps a support group or someone outside of the situation who has been through something similar. Good communication skills may not solve all of your problems, but learning to listen more effectively and voice your own thoughts, feelings, and needs in any given situation without creating further drama or disconnection is key to staying healthy and well through your caregiving experience. Keeping these conversations to yourself will negatively impact you and has the potential to come out in negative ways toward your client, patient, or loved one and also puts you at high risk for caregiver burnout.

CHAPTER FIVE

CAREGIVER BURNOUT

When the well's dry, we
know the worth of water."

—Benjamin Franklin

D o you feel worn out? Overextended? Tired all the time? If so, you're not alone. Balancing a busy personal and work life can feel virtually impossible, and then adding the responsibilities of caregiving to your already busy life can simply be too much. At first, you may think, *I can handle this*, but over time the extra responsibilities become overwhelming. In my work — both on myself and with my clients — I quickly realized that we all need to learn to genuinely start taking care of ourselves first. The fact is, you can't save anyone else until you learn to save yourself. So I would strongly suggest you learn to be a little more selfish, in a good way, so you can preserve yourself and stay healthy throughout your caregiving journey. Putting your needs first, learning to listen to your body, and taking care of yourself on all levels — mentally, physically, emotionally, and spiritually — will benefit you and your care recipient by making you a much better caregiver.

EXHAUSTION

Experiments conducted in the nineteenth century revealed that if you put a frog in hot water, it will jump out right away, but if you put the frog in tepid water and heat it up very gradually, it will not perceive the danger and will boil to death. These experiments have since been refuted, but it still serves as a useful metaphor for the inability or unwillingness of people to react to threats that arise gradually rather than suddenly.

Although I had jumped straight into the pot of boiling water without sticking a toe in (or a thermometer) to check the temperature, I can still compare myself to the frog in the sense that I was burning and didn't recognize the need to get out. I was feeling the heat but instead ignored the threat. I told myself to be strong. I didn't want to disappoint anyone or be perceived as incapable, incompetent, or weak. But the truth was I had no time to myself, I was not sleeping well, and my patience was wearing thin, not just with my grandmother, but also with my kids, my husband, and myself. Basically, I'd get up, get dressed, and go to work, only to come home after a full day to take over my responsibilities of caring for my kids and my grandmother until I collapsed into bed at the end of the day, only to do it all over again the next day. My husband and I were in similar boats, only our boats were drifting apart. We were both so very tired.

I did my best to put on my little happy face before walking out of the house every morning, and I appeared very successful from the outside, but on the inside, I was barely surviving.

"Life is busy, but I'm good," I'd respond when someone asked how I was doing. I did my best to hide the struggles, anxieties, self-doubt, guilt, fears, and other negative thoughts and emotions. I didn't ask for help, and I didn't want anyone to know I couldn't handle things — other than my husband, who helped carry the burden and meet all of the demands of this new role. With my grandmother now living with us, we were providing around-the-clock care and supervision. I was constantly worrying about things that were actually happening, as well as things that were not (but could possibly happen in the future). I was her power of attorney for personal care, in conjunction with my mother, and my husband was power of attorney for finances with my uncle. Since my mom and uncle were not around, my husband and I were attending to her every need, as well as the needs perceived by others.

"I talked to her on the phone last night. She didn't sound very good. I'm thinking you should make her a doctor's appointment."

"Is she eating well? She seems to be losing an awful lot of weight. Maybe you could look into meals on wheels?"

"Can you stop at the pharmacy and pick up her new medication?"

"Do you think she should be driving? This is the second time she's backed into a post. I'm really not sure it is safe for her to keep driving."

"She hasn't been showering, and I noticed she's always wearing the same clothes. Maybe she needs homecare."

"The tax bill needs to be paid."

A lot of people had a lot of opinions on what my grandmother needed, and I felt as though the complete burden of all these expectations and responsibilities was being piled on me. Everyone lived too far away to help, and I wasn't asking for help either. Instead, I tried to keep my head above the surface of the boiling water. Before I knew it, I was exhibiting the classic signs of caregiver burnout, including irritability, hopelessness, helplessness, anxiety, poor sleep, weight loss, withdrawing from family and friends, loss of interest in activities, fatigue, stress, low energy, and loss of motivation. I had started to rely on some negative coping strategies. My situation was definitely going from bad to worse.

PRACTICAL EXERCISE — DEALING WITH EXHAUSTION

Separate a sheet of paper into two columns. In the left-hand column, write all of your healthy ways of coping with your caregiving role and responsibilities. In the right-hand column, write all of your unhealthy ways of coping with them. Be thorough.

REFLECTIVE QUESTIONS

- On a scale of 1 to 5 (1 being least exhausted and 5 being most exhausted), how exhausted are you?

- Measuring by a specific number of weeks, how long have you been at this level of exhaustion?

- What do you think will happen if you don't deal with the factors contributing to your exhaustion? In other words, if nothing changes, where/how do you see yourself in six or twelve months from now?

BURNOUT

There are many definitions of caregiver burnout, but let's agree to use the following as a working definition: *Caregiver burnout is a state of mental, emotional, and physical exhaustion caused by caregiving over a prolonged period of time.*

Some have asked how caregiver burnout is different from depression. Specific diagnoses will be for your health professional to distinguish and determine, but I will say that the symptoms of caregiver burnout and depression are very similar, with the main difference being the cause. In other words, depression can be caused by many factors, whereas caregiver burnout is specifically caused by the chronic stress involved in the act of caregiving.

So how do you know if you're just tired, or if you're experiencing burnout? A good way to find out is to take a break for a few days. If you feel rejuvenated afterward, or if your symptoms resolve quickly after making positive adjustments to your caregiving situation, you're probably just tired and in need of a break or a change of pace. With burnout, your symptoms will continue and possibly worsen even after you've taken a good break, made significant changes to improve your caregiving situation, or even once it's over. For example, once I accepted that I could no longer care for my grandmother and she went to live in a nursing home, I thought life would return to normal. But it didn't. My negative thoughts and emotions were still there. I was exhausted and incapable of dealing with my day-to-day life, even after I was back to my normal duties. Even after taking care of and resolving the stresses involved in my caregiving situation.

What I'm about to share with you is my real-life experience with caregiver burnout. My intention is simply to provide a concrete example of how exhaustion left unaddressed can lead to burnout.

Since this was not my first breakdown or depression, I was surprised I didn't recognize the signs. I experienced my first depression in my teens, and then had a postpartum depression at twenty-four after the birth of my first child. I suppose I was so caught up in the rat race and in survival mode that I didn't see this one coming. There was just too much clutter and chaos going on in my mind. Too many things to do. Too much to keep up with. On good days, I could keep up the act. On bad days, everything was too overwhelming, and I didn't have the strength, energy, or willpower to deal with any of it. It was a struggle to get through the day. A struggle to accomplish even the smallest tasks. I started relying on old, unproductive coping mechanisms, even though I was thirty years old and a therapist — I knew better but for some reason couldn't bring myself to do better. I knew I should be making healthier choices and managing my stress better, but my energy was depleted and there was nothing left in my reserves. Then one day I went to work, and my boss called me to her office. She asked if I was okay, and I immediately broke down and told her how I'd been hanging on by a thread. She was supportive. She suggested I talk to my family physician and think about taking some time off work to take care of myself. What a blow that was! All along I thought I was hiding it well, but apparently I wasn't fooling anyone but myself.

PRACTICAL EXERCISE — COMPLETE A STRESS SELF-ASSESSMENT QUESTIONNAIRE

If you are wondering whether you are experiencing caregiver burnout, you probably are, and I would suggest you speak to your primary health care provider as soon as possible. If you don't think you're quite there yet, take the time to ask someone you trust for their opinion. If that's not an option, you can do the short stress survey in appendix B, which will give you a quick idea of where you're at.

REFLECTIVE QUESTIONS

- Have you noticed a decline in your mental or physical health (e.g., increased anxiety, irritability, insomnia, feelings of helplessness and hopelessness)?

- Are you experiencing relationship problems that you didn't have before (e.g., marital, family conflict, work conflicts, etc.)?

- Has anyone suggested you should slow down, take time off, or take better care of yourself? If so, what have you done about it?

SELF-CARE

Many people think it is selfish to put their own needs before someone else's. Before someone who needs them and depends on them. Many of us were taught to give freely to others and take care of other people's needs before our own. We see examples of this every day; every time a child is told to share their toys even as they are playing with them, when we are asked to consider the feelings of others without validating our own, when we are constantly asked to give a few dollars nearly every time we go out, even though we may be struggling to meet our own financial responsibilities. We do it because we don't want to say no. We don't want to look bad or like we don't care. So we give of ourselves, sometimes more than we have. We think we are doing the right thing; the "good" thing. But we are not! It is not healthy to give so much of ourselves that it depletes our own mental, emotional, and physical reserves. As much as I still believe it is important to give to others, I no longer believe we should give to the detriment of our own well-being. We must prioritize and take care of ourselves first and let go of the misconception that it is selfish.

I have learned the hard way that self-care is an absolute necessity. As a counsellor, I thought I knew all about "self-care," and when I finally realized I was having a burnout, my initial response was to eat more spinach, do yoga, go to the gym more often, make an appointment for a massage, hair, nails, etc. My understanding of self-care was simply to take more time to pamper myself and do "healthy" things. It turned out these were just more things to do, more appointments, more obligations, and more reasons to feel bad about myself when, for example, I skipped a workout. I have nothing against these methods of self-care and do believe we should all take time to do nice things for ourselves: a bath, listening to music, finding a healthy distraction. These are all great strategies that might make you feel better for a while, but these things alone are not going to provide a permanent solution or give you what you really need.

In order to develop real solutions so you can enjoy a balanced, healthy life while providing the level of care that feels good to you, the underlying reasons you are overextending yourself and taking on too much need to be examined and resolved. You may believe it's not fair to "unload" some of your duties onto someone else. You may feel guilty or worry that you will regret not being your loved one's "end-all-be-all" once they are gone. All these things may be true, but if you don't take charge of your own wellness now, you may not be able to care for your loved one at all as time goes on. Since I didn't know my own limits and expected more of myself than I was capable of under the circumstances, I became exhausted and consequently suffered burnout. From this experience, I have gained a real understanding of the saying, "If you don't take care of yourself, you can't take care of anyone else," and I also have a much deeper understanding of the true meaning of "self-care."

PRACTICAL EXERCISE — THINK ABOUT YOUR LIFE BEYOND CAREGIVING

This is a difficult step for many because we get so caught up in our caregiving roles and responsibilities that we forget who we are, what we value, and what brings a deep sense of joy to our lives. But it's time to rediscover yourself. Make a list of all the things you love to do (or used to love doing). If you've really lost touch with yourself, it may help to think about what made you happy as a child or how you used to spend your spare time before becoming a caregiver.

REFLECTIVE QUESTIONS

- What dreams did you put on hold because of your caregiving role and responsibilities?
- Beyond caregiving, what is most important in your life today?
- What would it take for you to be able to take care of your own needs as you move along your caregiving journey?

WHY WE GIVE TOO MUCH

There are different types of people in this world. Have you ever noticed that no matter what, some people will never be caregivers, regardless of the situation? Even if they are the last possible option, they will find a way out? They will send Mom to a nursing home without even thinking of taking her into their home, and without too much guilt. Are they selfish? Is it fair? I don't know, but do we need to judge them as being uncaring or self-centred? And why is it that we praise and reinforce people who are burning themselves out by giving more than they have? Is there a happy medium? I believe there is and that it is available to all of us. In order to find that balance, we must understand why we give too much in the first place.

During my caregiving experience, I was completely unaware that I was overcompensating for my feelings of inadequacy within my family. I wanted to please them and show them I was a good and worthy person. Your reasons for giving too much may be very different, but understand that if you are giving too much, an underlying belief is driving you.

When you think of other people in similar caregiving situations, you may find some are also taking on too much, while others are not taking on any caregiving duties at all, and yet some are taking on what they can handle and sharing the rest of the duties and responsibilities. In other words, not everyone feels, thinks, or behaves in the same ways when it comes to caregiving. But the question is… why?

To answer this question, think back to past caregiving situations you've experienced or observed and what thoughts you had about them. For example, did you have a saintly aunt who stayed by your grandma's side for fifteen years? Did everyone admire and praise this person? Did you have a bad-ass cousin who didn't come to weddings or funerals because he was too busy surfing in Japan? Did you judge him? Determining our judgements is a great indication of why we do what we do. Once you figure out who you are judging and what you are judging them for, and why, you will develop incredible insights into yourself and the reasons why you are giving too much. Also think about what you feel you are being judged about and/or judging yourself for.

Here are some examples of beliefs and judgements to help you consider what might be driving you to give too much.

EXAMPLES OF BELIEFS

"I grew up in a very religious household, and I can't tell you how many times I heard about how so-and-so won her place in Heaven by selflessly caring for someone else. As a child, it was made very clear to me that God favours those who give themselves up in service to others, no matter the cost to themselves. Those who didn't were basically going to Hell, as far as I could tell."

"I often heard my mother talking about how she had nothing but admiration for Aunt Mary, who was racking up good karma by selflessly taking care of her miserable sick husband."

"From the time I can remember, I was praised for being helpful. For thinking of others and doing good deeds. I realize now that in many ways I was helping others in order to meet my needs for attention and praise. This has led to overcaring and overhelping almost to the point of it being an addiction."

"I was taught that my own needs were not important. It was not so much in words, but in actions."

"*She's so strong, kind, caring, loving, patient, selfless* ... and the list of compliments aimed at people who were always there to help others quickly imprinted on my young mind the message that those who give freely of themselves, even if it's to the point of exhaustion, are judged positively by others."

EXAMPLES OF JUDGEMENTS

"What kind of wife would I be if I left my sick husband?"

"How would I feel if the roles were reversed?"

"How many sacrifices did my grandmother make for me when I was a child? Surely I can make some for her now."

"I can't imagine a parent placing their own disabled child in care. So heartless!"

"Now that he's dead, I bet she regrets not taking care of him while he was still here."

If you are giving too much of yourself, you need to start asking yourself why. What are your beliefs about caregiving? Where did they come from? And what are you getting out of it? In other words, what's in it for you being the family hero or the martyr? Are you being reinforced for giving too much through compliments and positive feedback from others? Was it something ingrained in you as a child that makes you believe it is good to give too much? Or are you simply concerned with what other people will think of you if you don't? Perhaps you feel you are intrinsically motivated to give, and this may be true, but if you're giving too much, there are certainly other factors at play.

There are many reasons why we give too much, and understanding these reasons will help you fulfill your caregiver role in a more responsible way that takes *you* and *your* needs into consideration. This, I have learned, is the most important piece of the self-care puzzle — putting your needs as a priority.

PRACTICAL EXERCISE

Take time to think about your beliefs about caregiving and reflect on where these beliefs came from. Journal about which of the statements above resonated most with you and why.

REFLECTIVE QUESTIONS

- Are you exceeding your limitations? If so, what beliefs are leading you to seek to accomplish things that are beyond your limitations?

- Is there someone you are trying to please or impress by doing too much? If so, who? And why?

- Were you rewarded for being selfless and for meeting everyone else's needs above your own? Or did you see someone else being rewarded for this? If so, by whom and for what, specifically?

CODEPENDENCE

In many caregiving situations, the caregiver and care recipient can start to lose their sense of identity and individuality. In other words, they become enmeshed. They lose the line between where one person ends and the other begins. This can initially meet the caregiver's need for importance or purpose, but it can lead to long-term problems in the relationship. On the care recipient's side, it can create a sense of learned helplessness, a feeling of worthlessness, and an imbalance in the relationship, as discussed in Chapter Three.

The classic definition of codependence has to do with control, nurturing, and enabling usually in a relationship that involves drug or alcohol dependence. For the purpose of this chapter, I am using the word codependence more loosely and in the context of doing for others what they can do for themselves as a way to feel a sense of purpose or a sense of control. When a loved one is diagnosed with a serious illness, we often don't know what to do. We turn to Dr. Google. We scare ourselves. We try to find ways to regain control over the situation. We have great intentions, and we do our best to meet the immediate needs of the care recipient, but we can do too much. More than they need us to do. We may treat our loved ones as though they are more fragile than they actually are and start taking away their opportunities to do things they are capable of doing. Perhaps it's quicker if we do it ourselves, or perhaps we just don't want to see them struggle. By taking over, both caregiver and care recipient fall into a pattern of over caring/overdoing and learned helplessness, respectively.

In most cases the care recipient does not want to be a burden. They do not want to lose their independence, and they still need to feel like they are making a contribution and have a purpose in life. Perhaps they can no longer contribute in the same ways they used to, but unless the person is on their deathbed or in a state where they truly cannot function at all, there are things they can do to contribute to their own care and possibly to yours. Remember, *everyone* needs a sense of purpose, some control, and meaning in their lives. By overcaring, you become the care recipient's handicap as well as your own. So if you are tired, exhausted, and possibly on the edge of burnout, seriously consider whether you are doing things you don't need to be and whether there are things your care recipient could do for themselves.

This will restore your care recipient's sense of independence to a degree and promote more balance in the relationship, while relieving you of the burden of doing too much.

You may think you're the only one who can take care of your loved one, and that may be true, but if it is true, it does beg the question of who will take over their care if you are burnt out and can't do it anymore.

PRACTICAL EXERCISE — BREAK CODEPENDENT PATTERNS

Watch the YouTube video, *Breakthrough with Tony Robbins, Episode 1*, with Frank and Kristen Alioto. In this video, Tony helps a couple who experienced a serious tragedy on their wedding night. Overnight, Frank became a quadriplegic and Kristen became his nurse. Watch how this couple went from a state of burnout, depression, and codependence to taking their lives back and getting their relationship back on track. Perhaps this situation will not reflect yours, but it will inspire you to think of ways to get out of any overcaring patterns. If possible, watch the episode with your care recipient and have an honest conversation afterward about any insights either of you may have gained.

REFLECTIVE QUESTIONS

- What parts of your life can you take back? What parts of your loved one's life can you help them take back?
- What limitations have you been putting on yourself and on your loved one?
- How can you empower your care recipient instead of enabling them?

ME FIRST

My breakdown opened my eyes and showed me everything I was taking for granted. The path I was on, caring for everyone else before myself, led me to the brink of losing everything. I had lost the connection in my marriage because I was too busy trying to meet my own unrealistic expectations and commitments. My energy was depleted. I had nothing left for him, or at least, not enough. My job was suffering. My kids. My own physical and mental health. Caregiver burnout in many other cases (but not all) can be a result of a lack of responsibility you've taken toward yourself. Sometimes it is code for "I'm not taking care of myself and my own needs."

My biggest takeaway from my caregiving experience is that I am responsible for taking care of me first. In my conversations with my new husband, we talk about how we can love and care for each other in a way that is as free of burden and resentment as possible, and in a way that allows us to take care of ourselves first and foremost. I believe I will again take on a caregiver role in someone's life, but because of what I've learned, I will do so in a way that honours my own wishes, needs, values, and goals and allows them to maintain as much independence, control, and purpose as possible.

PRACTICAL EXERCISE — GOAL-SETTING

What is your current reality? Where do you want to be? Where are you going in life? By looking at the different areas of your life and asking yourself these questions, you can start to get clarity on what goals *you* want to achieve. On a sheet of paper, write the following six headings: Financial, Emotional, Physical, Spiritual, Professional, Relationships. For each of these categories, write what you want to achieve in the next six to twelve months. Be specific, and make sure your goals are measurable. For example, if you want to lose weight, include your exact target weight, by what date you want to achieve it, and the specific methods for how you plan to achieve this goal. Note: Keep these goals handy, because you will need them again in Chapter Six.

REFLECTIVE QUESTIONS

- Imagine yourself having completed each one of your goals and imagine how you will feel.

- What specific thoughts and actions will you need to take on a daily basis in order to align yourself with this goal (for each goal separately)?

- How will you know when you've achieved your goals?

REACHING OUT

I talked about this already, and it may seem redundant, but the reason for this is that reaching out for help can be one of the toughest parts for many caregivers, as well as *the* most important when it comes to preserving your own mental, emotional, and physical wellness while on your caregiving journey. Removing our egos from the equation and realizing we cannot do this alone, and *should* not do it alone, is a healthy starting point. Reaching out is not a weakness. In fact, I would suggest *not* reaching out is the weakness.

When you muster the courage to ask for help, and once others know what you need help with (specific tasks), you will likely find that most are willing to assist you and your loved one. You may think it's wrong to put your responsibilities on someone else, but just think of the satisfaction you have felt when you were able to help someone in need, and you genuinely wanted to. Then look at the flip side and think of how it felt when you genuinely wanted to help someone and they wouldn't accept your help.

Don't rob people of their opportunity to be there for you in your times of need, since it usually gives them great pleasure, especially if they can help in ways that tap into their own areas of strength and expertise. For example, if your sister is a great cook, perhaps she can take over responsibility for needs related to cooking or food. If Uncle Joe loves driving, perhaps he can take over driving his brother for out-of-town appointments. When I finally reached out for help because I had no choice, my uncle gladly took over many of the financial responsibilities. My mom said she had been thinking of moving back to help out, and she did so shortly afterward. My aunt also helped in whatever ways she could (she lived in Whitehorse). Here I was feeling resentful as I imagined my family members relaxing on their sofas thinking up more and more tasks to add to my to-do list, but when I finally broke down and reached out for help, I realized my family wanted to help. The criticism and expectations I had perceived from them were not accurate; they were actually feeling helpless, and it was their way of showing concern and doing their best to support their mother from a distance.

In a caregiving situation recently recounted to me, a caregiver reached out to her brothers for help, and although they did not feel capable of providing direct care, both offered to pay a monthly amount for some professional home care services. She felt good about this arrangement, and they were also happy to be able to make a contribution that didn't involve bathing and toileting their father.

I want to make it crystal clear that reaching out is not about letting people know how much of a jerk they've been for not figuring out that you needed help. It's about letting them know where you are at right now and how you've been affected by the situation. It's about getting specific about what you need. When I approached my family, I told them where I was at. That I was experiencing burnout. That the responsibilities of caring for my grandmother were too much. I explained why I hadn't asked for more help, including the fact that I didn't always know what I needed help with and didn't want to be seen as a failure. I didn't point fingers. I just explained my challenges as best as I understood them myself and told them I needed help. Together we figured out how they could lend a hand.

Most of us find it hard to reach out, but if you are a caregiver, learning to ask for help and learning to say yes to what is offered will make this journey so much easier in the long run. It's one thing to deal with a short-term crisis, or a short-term caregiving situation, but if you are going to be in this for the long haul, you will need to develop a plan for how you will take care of yourself by getting the support you need to get your own goals and priorities back to the forefront of your life.

PRACTICAL EXERCISE — PUT YOUR HELPERS TO WORK

Assuming you've already completed the practical exercises in previous chapters, including setting up a care plan, brainstorming with family members and friends, and enlisting help, as well as tapping into community resources, you are well on your way to creating the time and energy to meet your own mental, emotional, and physical needs. If you haven't set up a care plan for your loved one, do so as soon as possible. If you haven't enlisted help, get on it. People may shy away if they don't really know what you're asking of them. But if you give them a specific task, one they feel comfortable with, they will likely be happy to help. When someone asks how they can help, instead of saying, "I'm fine, I've got this on my own," thank them for asking and show them the list of duties they could help with. Ask if there is something on the list that interests them and if it's something they could pitch in with on a regular basis. Maybe they can bring a meal once a week, help clean the house every two weeks, or perhaps they could occasionally offer transportation to a doctor's appointment.

REFLECTIVE QUESTIONS

- Make a list of the top five things that make your caregiving experience a challenge.

- Is there anyone who may be willing and able to take on some of your more challenging caregiving responsibilities?

- If you reached out for help, what would you have more time and energy for? In other words, what could you do to take care of yourself if you had more time and energy?

CONCLUSION

After my burnout, my grandmother went into a nursing home. I was no longer able to care for her, and no one else was able to take over her care, since her needs had increased exponentially as her disease progressed. The truth was, she was no longer safe. She had started to wander and do other dangerous things such as crossing busy streets in traffic, leaving the oven on or the water running, etc. The transition to the nursing home was initially very difficult. My grandmother had worked for the local newspaper her entire adult life, and she reminded me that she knew important people. She threatened to call the media and tell them what I was doing to her. It was truly heart-wrenching.

But lo and behold, a week after she moved in, she discovered she enjoyed it at the nursing home. She talked about how great it was that she didn't have to cook or clean or do laundry (not that she'd been doing any of that stuff). She also enjoyed having company and said everyone was so nice to her. In addition, my family felt reassured she was safe and that I wasn't being burdened with all of the responsibilities. I thought, *Wow, are you kidding me?* All this time, I was thinking I was the "hero," but that turned out to be far from the truth. Up until that point, I truly thought I'd been doing her a great service, but I couldn't help but wonder if I would have been a much better caregiver all along had she gone to the nursing home in the first place. Once she was there, I felt reassured that she was being well taken care of.

I visited her regularly, took her out for walks and out for lunch at her favourite restaurant (Wendy's). I wasn't stressed or resentful anymore. I started asking questions and listening more. Although she had lost her short-term memory, she loved telling me stories about her childhood; how she would play hockey or latch on to car bumpers in the winter for a ride, or how she used to run the logs and jump off the old bridges into the river. She would light up as she told me about going out with her father on horse and buggy to make dairy deliveries, how they got treated to the leftover ice cream, how she learned to speak and understand French — things I never knew about her. I started to learn about who she was as a person before she even became a grandmother to me. I had so much more patience with her. I started to enjoy my time with her, even though she didn't always know who I was and still repeated the same questions and stories over and over again. When I felt I was starting to get frustrated with the repetition,

I would kiss her goodbye and let her know that I'd see her again soon. I felt good about our interaction, knowing I didn't have to worry about her every waking hour. She would remain safe and sound until I saw her next. She would walk me to the door and wave goodbye to the "nice lady" who had kindly come to visit her. Although she no longer knew my name and usually didn't recognize me as her grandchild, I always felt she knew I was someone special to her.

As you can imagine, making drastic changes to my caregiving situation was very difficult at first. I felt like a failure, like I was letting everyone down. Like I was hurting my grandmother. But I have since realized the impact of the negative energy I was bringing to the relationship and how my resentment was affecting us both (and other areas of my life). In the long run, making these changes to my caregiving situation allowed us to restore a positive and loving relationship. It ultimately saved our relationship and saved me.

CHAPTER SIX

CONSCIOUS CAREGIVING

"First enlightenment,
then the laundry."

—Zen Proverb

t is a given that someone who is mentally, emotionally, physically, and spiritually taking care of
themselves will be a much better caregiver. As
the title suggests, conscious caregiving is about
becoming consciously aware — aware of ourselves,
of our relationships, of our pasts, and of how we are
relating and responding to what is going on in and
around us. This chapter is not only about becoming a
more conscious caregiver, but also about becoming a
more conscious human being in all aspects of life. With
enhanced self-awareness and heightened consciousness, you can learn to relax, accept the present moment,
and enjoy your experiences more fully. This conscious
awareness grows as you learn to pause and mindfully
notice the experiences you are having as an objective
observer, as opposed to being caught up in the hamster
wheel in your mind, racing around and around in an
endless cycle. It is recognizing that your caregiving
experience is just an experience. There is nothing factual
about it other than the fact you are having an experience. All the rest is your perception, interpretation, and
the meaning you've been attaching to it. And remember,
no matter what the experience, however positive or
negative, there will still be laundry to do!

THE BIGGER PICTURE

When we can pull ourselves up and above the events of our lives and
observe these experiences from a detached perspective, we can start to see
ourselves and our lessons in life far beyond what we are experiencing in any
particular moment. This caregiving experience, like all other experiences

124

that have made up the story of your life, is simply an experience to help you learn and evolve. Whether positive or negative, this experience will help you in ways you cannot yet imagine, as long as you stay open to the lessons. For example, I had no idea my caregiving experience would lead to writing a book about it fifteen years later. I never imagined I'd get over all the guilt and shame and actually be able to use this "negative" caregiving experience for such "positive" purposes. If someone would have looked into a crystal ball and told me that going through a burnout would be a turning point in my life that would allow me to positively impact others in such a massive way, I never would have believed it. I couldn't see the higher purpose — the bigger picture — but when I learned to rise above the content of my life and gain awareness of my own mental traps, I gained access to my higher lessons.

PRACTICAL EXERCISE — LOOK AT THE BIGGER PICTURE

Whether you are having a mostly positive or mostly negative caregiving experience, take the time to consider some of the lessons you might be learning from it. To do this, close your eyes and imagine yourself floating above your entire life, starting at the beginning. When you get to the start of your caregiving journey, fly very slowly over your caregiving experience. Stay high above it all. Keeping your bird's-eye view and detached perspective, see if you can identify some of the benefits. When you get to difficult parts, ask yourself, "What are the lessons here?"

Once you have completed this exercise, take a few minutes to read Paulo Coelho's short story, "The Lost Horse." (Google it!) Consider journaling about your reactions and any feelings that the story brought up for you.

REFLECTIVE QUESTIONS

- What benefits have resulted so far from your caregiving experience?
- If this experience had not been part of your life story, what positive experiences might you have missed out on?
- In what ways have you been able to use your caregiving experience to make a positive contribution to others (or how might you see yourself doing so in the future)?

THE BOX

To gain access to the bigger picture, it is helpful to recognize the smaller picture, or what I like to call "The Box." When I was nineteen, I had a short glimpse of enlightenment. It was a very difficult period in my life, and I'll never forget around that same time, in one of my philosophy classes, learning about Plato's "Allegory of the Cave". This story contributed in a significant way to my fleeting moment of enlightenment. Plato's story describes prisoners who lived their lives chained up in a cave, facing a blank wall. As things pass between the cave opening behind them and a fire behind it, they can see shadows being cast on the wall in front of them. They start to label these shadows and tell stories about them. They believe these shadows to be reality instead of the projections they actually are. When the prisoners are finally freed, they come to realize the shadows were not reality at all, as they'd once thought. They now understood that their "reality" was manufactured by their own minds based on their misperceptions and misinterpretations as reflected by their very limited view from inside "The Box."

We must understand this is all part of the human condition, to be tethered by our perceptions and interpretations, no matter how absurd they may be. When we escape from our box, we gain a whole new perspective and find a new world that would be completely incomprehensible to us if we were still imprisoned in the box. From this new "reality," we can reinterpret *everything*. We can discover a new meaning and purpose to the ups, the downs, the twists and turns, the victories and defeats, and all of the adventures and moments that make up our lives. When we are able to take an objective perspective and rise above the content of our lives, we can see things in an entirely different light.

PRACTICAL EXERCISE — REINTERPRET YOUR STORY

Every event has countless interpretations. Choose a recent "negative" event from your caregiving experience and write out every possible interpretation, no matter how silly or unlikely it may seem. Once you've brainstormed all possibilities, choose the interpretation that would serve you best.

REFLECTIVE QUESTIONS

Using the event from the practical exercise above, answer the following questions:

- If you had a big-picture view, how might you see this event differently?
- What could be the higher lessons in this experience?
- How might this experience benefit you, or others, in the long run?

MENTAL AWARENESS

Do you know what's going on in your mind on a moment-to-moment basis? Do you know the average person has something like 70,000 thoughts per day? This number is shocking, but it also validates why we feel like there is constant chatter going on in our minds. *Kapicitta* is the Buddhist term sometimes used to describe this constant chatter. Kapicitta can be translated as "monkey mind"; it is when our mind jumps from thought to thought like a monkey jumps from tree to tree. Mental awareness is the state of being consciously aware of all of these thoughts and gaining the ability not to get attached to any of them.

After my burnout, my counsellor suggested I get away for a few days. He gave me specific instructions: "Go sit with your own mind and really pay attention to the thoughts that come up. What's tripping you up is all happening between your own two ears, and it's time to find out what that is. Bring a journal and a pen. Nothing else."

I hesitated. I had no idea how spending a few days on my own with only a pen and paper — no phone, no books, no TV, no access to the outside world — could help. But I was suffering. And I trusted him. So I did it. I spent four days alone in a room with my journal, getting out only to go to the bathroom next to my room (my friend brought meals in twice a day without looking at me or saying a peep). The door closed behind me, and I sat on the bed. With nothing to do and nothing to distract me, I started observing my mind carefully. Prior to this experience, I thought I had a pretty good sense of what was going through my mind on a daily basis. Boy, was I wrong! I was shocked when I actually discovered what was happening in there. I was so used to just jumping on whatever negativity train was going by that I no longer even noticed when I was on it. All the self-destructive thoughts were like popcorn popping in my brain — and it was about everything: *I am not good enough. Smart enough. Pretty enough. What's wrong with me? Why can't I just be happy? I'm a bad person, mother, daughter, sister, wife, employee, caregiver.* The list went on and on. With every thought, I felt worse and worse, and I was only a couple of hours into this "retreat." I thought, *I am not going to survive four days with myself.*

As I paid close attention and got brutally honest about the repetitive stories that were playing out in my mind, I quickly discovered that my mind was my worst enemy. It was like my mind had been infected with a virus. The same way cancer spreads and kills healthy cells, my negative, self-destructive thoughts had taken root and were destroying whatever healthy thoughts I might have once had. I realized I had to turn this around, and quickly.

PRACTICAL EXERCISE — OBSERVE YOUR MIND

We become so used to listening to the voice in our heads and believing everything it says that we often don't even notice it slowly poisoning us. Before we can learn to turn it off (or at least change the channel), we must first notice what it is saying. Start listening to the voice in your head, because how you think will dictate how you feel. You can flood yourself with positive thoughts or negative thoughts, but remember, your emotions will follow your thoughts. So take five minutes today to do a simple mindfulness exercise. All you need to do is practice watching your thoughts for five minutes without getting involved in them. When a thought arises, label it and allow it to pass through your consciousness. If you notice you've gotten caught up in thoughts, bring your awareness back to your breathing. Concentrate on the inflow and outflow of your breath. Then try to spend five minutes with your care recipient in a total state of mindfulness, where you simply pay attention with presence to what is going on in the moment.

REFLECTIVE QUESTIONS

- What thoughts do you keep getting caught up in?
- Are your thoughts in alignment with the caregiving experience you want to have?
- What was it like to spend five minutes in complete presence with your care recipient?

PAST CONDITIONING

Past conditioning sets us up to view experiences in certain ways, but it doesn't mean what we perceive and interpret as true is actually "The Truth."

All this time, I had been buying into my own stories about myself, about others, and about how the world works. I was thinking my problems were all out there in the world, and I was blaming my husband, my job, my past, my caregiving responsibilities, and anything I could think of. But here I was waking up to the fact that my "reality" wasn't as real or as true as I had thought it to be. I was finally recognizing the need to strip away the old mental conditioning that was no longer serving me. It was time to break through my black sheep story, my failure story, my abandonment story, and all the other stories that were affecting my ability to be a more conscious caregiver and more conscious human being. Some of these stories were based on my own misperceptions and misinterpretations, and others had been passed down to me from the adults in my life when I was just a little girl, probably around the same time I was led to believe in Santa Claus, the Easter Bunny, and the Tooth Fairy — when I was open to believing anything. Eventually, I learned these characters were fictional, but all the other stuff continued to run in the background of my life, affecting me in ways I had absolutely no awareness of.

For the most part, people live their lives like programmed robots, but we need to break free from this programming if it's not working for us. The mind is a very powerful tool, but if you're a slave to it, it can quickly take over and bring you down the wrong path. We have all been conditioned, and when we are not really aware of the stuff we are facilitating for ourselves, we keep living into it. The truth is, the past can never change, but the meaning you attached to your past experiences can. Once you are able to successfully remove the meaning from an experience, it just doesn't matter any more.

Understand that for everything stopping you from going forward, there's something behind pulling you back. It's like having a rope attached to your waist, and every time you build up momentum, these past challenges and/ or past conditioning pull you back. Unfortunately, most people create a world based on the script that was given to them, and they stay in "The Box" their entire lives. They find people who will help keep them in their act and help them play out the same movie over and over again, much like *Groundhog Day*. When you start to uncover and unravel the stories that are running rampant in your mind and start peeling back the layers of how your thinking is creating the same situations over and over again, you will start to recognize that you are the main character in your life, and *you* are the only one that can change the script you've been living to. Once you break out of these old mental and emotional patterns and stop believing the past scripts that were passed down to you, you can put an end to the painful experiences from your past. At this point you will become a more conscious human being, and with this heightened level of consciousness, you will also become a better caregiver.

After about two days of sitting in absolute boredom, with nothing to do but watch the repetitive stories running in my mind, I finally realized nothing was going to change until *I* changed it. As long as I kept playing the same movie reels in my mind, the same "reality" would continue to be projected onto the screen in front of me. That was when I made the decision to invest in thinking different and being different in my own world, because the truth is, you can never get away from *you*. No matter how far you move or where you go, the voice in your head will still be there. Regardless of how much you change your outside environment, if the inside always looks and sounds the same, in time, your mind will recreate on the outside what's playing out on the inside. For example, if you are rushing and impatient in your mind with thoughts racing a hundred miles an hour, you will likely be rushing and impatient with your care recipient. Or like me, if you have a failure story running in the background, you will be caregiving for the wrong reasons or giving too much of yourself as a way to prove your worth.

PRACTICAL EXERCISE — TAME YOUR INNER VOICE

Start treating your mind like a wild horse. Start observing it, watching its patterns, approaching it slowly, and making friends with it. With firmness and patience, the horse will be tamed, and there you have it: a partner for life. My experience shows that if you don't commit to this, you will continue to be dragged around like a rag doll, holding on to a rope behind your wild and crazy horse, taking all the bumps and bruises. We all need to start being our own best friend and work to eliminate all self-defeating thoughts. You only have this one you, and no matter who you're with, where you go, or what you do, *you* are still there. The voice in your head follows you no matter where you are, so you may as well start making friends with yourself!

Your exercise today is to stand in front of a mirror at least ten times, look yourself in the eye and say, "I love you. It's you and me until the end. I got you. You are safe." You can change the wording as long as it is a loving message acknowledging that you are getting in touch with your inner voice and being gentle with yourself.

REFLECTIVE QUESTIONS

For every thought you have, ask yourself:

- Is this true? Is it helpful?
- Are these thoughts/beliefs your own, or did someone else pass them on to you?
- Would you say the things you're saying to yourself to your best friend, a client, or to your care recipient?

COMMITMENT AND DISCIPLINE

The commitment to changing my thoughts and the meaning I had attached to certain experiences was a huge discipline. Just catching my negative thoughts was hard, because I was so used to believing them. They seemed so natural to me at the time. So, for many months after I made my decision to change my thoughts, I wore an elastic band around my wrist and snapped it every time those negative, self-defeating thoughts entered my mind, and I'd say: *I don't believe you, that's not true, this isn't real.* Sometimes they'd go away, but other times they came right back with a vengeance, so I'd journal about them. I'd get them out of my head. I wrote about opposite thoughts and how I would feel if I believed those thoughts instead. I wrote until my mind was empty. This discipline took the thoughts out of my mind and put them on a piece of paper.

I wrote every day for years. Getting those thoughts out of my mind created a space within me — a space I could fill with more positive and productive thoughts. For example, one day I had been very impatient with my grandmother and had said to her, "Just stop talking, please," in a mean and elevated tone. I immediately felt terrible about it and apologized, but I couldn't let it go. Hours later, I was still beating myself up over my harsh reaction. So I sat down and started journaling about the repetitive and demeaning thoughts that were going through my mind. Things like: "I know it's not her fault, why do I always have to be so mean?" or "Why can't I just be more patient?" or "I'm a terrible caregiver," or "she'd be better off without me," etc. Once I got *all* of the negative thoughts out of my head, I started questioning them one by one. For example, was it true that I was always mean? Was I really a *terrible* caregiver? etc. Once I got all that negative stuff out of my head, there was a space to fill it with more positive thoughts, ones that would help me create a more positive internal environment for myself. This allowed me to be more kind and loving toward myself and in turn toward my grandmother.

When you make the commitment to keep the thoughts that have been haunting you out of your mind, you will need to be disciplined about it, because your mind will trick you into going back into habitual thought patterns, regardless of whether they are helpful or not.

PRACTICAL EXERCISE — ALIGN YOUR THOUGHTS AND ACTIONS WITH WHAT YOU WANT

Make a list of all of your goals related to your role as a caregiver (e.g., to be more patient, more relaxed, take better care of yourself, etc.). Then for each goal, consider whether your current thinking is in alignment with your goal. If you discover that your thinking is not in alignment with your goal, turn each of those thoughts into positive affirmations/ statements that will support you in achieving your goal. Write these affirming thoughts on Post-It notes and stick them everywhere as reminders.

REFLECTIVE QUESTIONS

- In what ways are your thoughts, feelings, and actions in alignment with your goals as a caregiver?

- What low-level thoughts (defined as thoughts that are not supporting you in your caregiving goals) are you still having?

- What is preventing you from eliminating your low-level thoughts?

SELF-AFFIRMATION SCRIPTS

Journaling is one great way to get negative, unproductive thoughts out of your mind, and positive self-affirmation scripts are a perfect way to replace them. Self-affirmation scripts are consciously chosen statements used to replace the inner scripts you've been repeating to yourself — all those things that are going around in your mind, based on your past conditioning, self-limiting decisions, and old mental patterns. Positive self-affirmations are a very powerful way to help align yourself with your goals by repro-gramming your unconscious mind quickly and effectively. When creating self-affirmation scripts, it is important to be as specific as possible without using any negatives. For example, if you say, "I don't want to get frustrated" or "I want to stop getting frustrated," there is a negative twist, so instead, keep it positive by saying something like, "I want to be more patient." These word choices may seem unimportant to you, but to your subconscious mind they are quite significant. Simple word choices can sabotage your success. For example, words like "try," "but," "maybe," or "if" can unconsciously trap you in unproductive mental patterns. The mind can be very sneaky, and retraining it will require creativity and conscious effort on your part. Here are some examples of self-affirmations scripts:

Example #1: I am confident and happy now because I am easily on track to achieving my goal of feeling more peace and calm in my life. I am easily able to balance the demands of caregiv-ing with other parts of my life. I realize that stress helps me in many ways and that managing my mental and emotional state is allowing me to use stress more positively and productively in my role as a caregiver. I am in a good place mentally, emotion-ally, and physically because I have learned how to manage my mind and my emotions. Now that I have released the pressures, expectations, and demands I was placing on myself, I feel more energized and am really able to enjoy life, and I feel like I can easily become a more conscious caregiver.

Example #2: I am confident and happy now because I am easily on track to achieving my goal of being a more confident and patient caregiver. I feel more peace and calm in my life now that I am journaling and taking time every day for myself. I am happy now because I am easily on track to achieving my goal of meeting my own needs. I realize that paying attention to what I want and need allows me to be a better caregiver.

Example #3: I feel great because I am spiritually connected to myself and to the people who matter to me. I am committed to seeing the good in myself and accepting self-love. I am happy, energized, and at my best now that I have established consistent habits to stay physically, emotionally, and spiritually healthy. I am a great caregiver now that I am loving myself and taking care of ME first!

Example #4: I am secure and at peace because I can easily balance the demands of my new caregiving role with the other aspects of my life. I am easily able to achieve work-life balance and feel calm and relaxed. Maintaining consistent healthy mental and physical habits is allowing me to be the best caregiver I can be.

PRACTICAL EXERCISE — CREATE A SELF-AFFIRMATION SCRIPT

Based on the goals you set for yourself in chapter five, create a self-affirmation script such as in the examples above that incorporates as many of your goals as possible. Once you've created your script, record it on your phone in a very melodic tone. Listen to your script as you're going to sleep every night, preferably with earphones. For quicker results, listen to it in the morning as well.

REFLECTIVE QUESTIONS

- How has your mind worked against you?
- In what other ways can you get your mind working for you?
- How will a more positive mindset affect your caregiving relationship?

GET A COACH

If you're asking: *Why does this keep happening to me?* then there is something in your past that needs resolution, and you will likely need help getting through it. These challenges won't go away on their own. They will just keep resurfacing in different ways until you can find someone who can really challenge you on the things you keep spinning around in. Someone who can challenge you to think differently. Someone who has the tools to pull you out of your story and help you get over the wall you keep getting stuck at. This person can be a friend, counsellor, or life coach, as long as it is someone you trust and someone who has the ability to be honest with you, and from whom you can accept it. Most importantly, it must be someone who has experience with the types of challenges you are dealing with. A lot of people are out there trying to help others when they haven't done their own work. If a coach is not walking what they're talking, they won't be able to help you get past the challenges that are holding you back. You will recognize the ones who walk what they talk because they won't be telling you the things you want to hear. Instead, they will be saying things you've likely never heard before. They will quickly and easily help you cut through your own stories and help you look at the stuff you've been avoiding. Going this deep may not be appealing to some people. Some may prefer to avoid their difficult experiences and deny the effect they are still having, but unless you're willing to open the vault and fully explore and expose the hidden aspects of yourself, you will remain in the same box, and your full mental and emotional capacity will remain dormant.

Let me forewarn you ... there is a real discomfort and vulnerability required in allowing someone to call you on your own stuff. And you might be shocked when you start to realize within yourself how much BS you've been telling yourself and how you've managed to find people who have that same kind of conditioning and who are willing to keep you in it. This is about getting back to the essence of who you are before you were stressed about caregiving, before you accepted self-limiting beliefs about yourself, before all the events and experiences that caused you to feel afraid, angry, resentful, sad, or guilty. If you're serious about getting in touch with who you really are, get a coach who will hold you accountable to the disciplines required to be a conscious caregiver and conscious human being.

We all want to get through these old challenges so we can experience happiness and freedom from within ourselves. When we truly go back and resolve these old challenges, they never show up again. But in order to get to the core of your issues, someone has to ask the tough questions. If you're willing to hear and work through those tough questions and resolve old challenges and issues, you can start living in freedom and reaping the benefits and rewards of your caregiving experience.

PRACTICAL EXERCISE — GET A COACH

It's normal to be blind to our own dysfunctional patterns and how they contribute to the repetitive problems in our lives, so getting a coach to help you recognize your mental and emotional patterns and to teach you how to break free from them is vital.

REFLECTIVE QUESTIONS

- Do you reach out when you are having a hard time with your caregiving situation? If so, to whom do you reach out, and can they pull you out of your spin?
- Who in your life can really challenge you to think differently?
- Who in your life can challenge you on your behaviour?

CONCLUSION

Being fully present with someone else requires us to be fully present and still within ourselves. If you want to develop a conscious approach to caregiving, you will need to learn to be more conscious within yourself. Once you do, you will find yourself feeling much better on the inside — happier, calmer, more patient — and projecting these positive feelings externally. Your care recipient will notice, as will everyone around you. They will see and feel the changes in you. Everyone will benefit from you becoming more consciously aware, especially you!

CHAPTER SEVEN

LIFE AFTER CAREGIVING

"From caring comes courage."

—Lao Tzu

As a caregiver, you have devoted a lot of time and energy to meeting the needs of your care recipient. Therefore, when your caregiving journey ends, it can be very difficult and can leave you feeling confused, disoriented, and lost. You may be wondering who you are and what to do with yourself. The way your caregiving journey ended will affect how you react and respond to this change in your life. For instance, if caregiving ended because your loved one passed away, your experience will be much different than if your loved one made a full recovery or someone else took over their care. These factors, as well as many others, will significantly impact how you move forward after your caregiving journey ends. Even if it hasn't yet come to an end, this chapter will help prepare you for when that time comes, as well as provide you with strategies to achieve and maintain an optimum state of wellness. Throughout this chapter, I have included quotes from the accompanying *Caregiving Insights* to reinforce important concepts and introduce you to the powerful messages from these inspirational authors.

READJUSTING TO LIFE

Just as your life changed drastically when your caregiving journey began, so it will change drastically when it ends. In my case, I went through two "endings." The first was when my grandmother went to live in a nursing home. I immediately went from being her primary caregiver, responsible for almost everything, to being a secondary caregiver with a fraction of the responsibilities. Plus, not long after she moved to the nursing home, my mother moved back to our hometown and took over all of the remaining caregiving responsibilities. I was no longer needed. It was disorienting, to say the least, but since I was recovering from caregiver burnout, it allowed me to refocus my time and energy and put myself as a priority. My mom stayed for about two years before going back out west. By that time, I had fully recovered and was ready to assist with my grandmother's care again. However, there weren't many caregiving duties remaining, because she was living in the secure dementia unit by this time. When my grandmother passed away two years later, the adaptation to life after caregiving was not nearly as difficult.

No matter how your caregiving journey ended, you may find it difficult to readjust to different schedules, new routines, and to life in general. Things don't just go back to normal once you shift out of your caregiving role. Sure, certain responsibilities may be lifted, but a sense of destabilization can be expected, especially after a long-term caregiving journey. You may feel as though you've lost your sense of purpose or even your identity. You may be tempted to run out and help someone else or find another distraction, but I would suggest you lean into the discomfort and give yourself some time to adjust and get through the barrage of emotions you can expect to experience. Don't make any big decisions during this period unless you have to. Things that might make perfect sense in your current state may not make sense later.

PRACTICAL EXERCISE — TAKE A BREAK

Lower your expectations of yourself and take it easy for a while. On the outside, it may seem like you have fewer demands and fewer things to do, but there is actually a major reorganization going on inside of you. So be very gentle with yourself during this adjustment period.

REFLECTIVE QUESTIONS

- How can you be gentler with yourself as you go through this adjustment period?
- How can you refocus the time and energy you were putting into your caregiving role and direct it back to yourself?
- How can you find mental and emotional healing?

GRIEF AND LOSS

When a caregiving journey ends because the care recipient passed away, there will be a much different grieving process than if the person made a full recovery or care was transferred to someone else. Even if your loved one is doing well, you may find yourself experiencing a huge sense of loss. If your caregiving role started long ago or occupied a lot of your time and energy — even if it took a huge toll on you — grief will be one of the many feelings you experience. It is important to give yourself permission to grieve your caregiving role. Understand there is no set timeframe for grieving, and this can vary quite significantly from person to person and from situation to situation. In my case, when my caregiving role ended the first time, there was a huge void. I felt I had lost my sense of purpose and a big part of my identity, whereas the final ending to my caregiving journey was much easier because it had been a gradual process of letting go. I had been able to enjoy a long, loving goodbye, and appreciate that my grandmother was no longer suffering. Again, I will say grieving is a very individual process, and many factors will affect the intensity, duration, and recovery period. It is such a complex emotional process that I have decided to write my next book on the topic of grief and loss.

PRACTICAL EXERCISE — GIVE YOURSELF PERMISSION TO GRIEVE

As mentioned previously, there is no single way to grieve or set duration to get through the grieving process. In fact, I would suggest you give yourself full permission to grieve for several months. During this period, honour your feelings and refrain from telling yourself things like: "I should be over this by now" or "I shouldn't feel this way." If after giving yourself permission to grieve, you feel you are not recovering or feeling worse rather than better as time goes on, reach out for help. Find someone who can help you move through your grieving process. By the same token, give yourself permission not to grieve or to take breaks from grieving. When my grandmother passed, I was not very sad and started wondering if something was wrong with me. I didn't realize my grieving process had happened over a period of six years, and I was already emotionally complete with her passing by the time she died. Therefore, if you're not grieving, that's okay too. Or if you simply need to take a time-out on grieving, give yourself permission to do that.

REFLECTIVE QUESTIONS

As you move through your grieving process, you can ask the following questions as suggested by Karen Hourtevenko in her chapter, "How to Manage Guilt and Grief":

- Is holding on to this grief helping me or holding me back?
- What advice would I give a friend if they were going through grief?
- What positive impact did the person you lost have on you?

FREEDOM AND RELIEF

Caregivers often set aside their own lives to care for someone else, so when that person no longer needs care, the caregiver may experience a sense of relief. That's not to say there is not a sense of grief as well, but simply that there can be a huge sense of relief in being released from your caregiving responsibilities. If the care recipient has passed on, the caregiver often feels relieved that their loved one is no longer suffering and is finally at rest. Most caregivers experience this sense of relief but also feel bad for feeling this way. The fact is, caregiving often takes us away from our own life pursuits, and the end of caregiving means we are getting our freedom back. Bonnie Mulvihill highlights the sense of relief that many caregivers experience when their caregiving journey comes to an end:

> I did not feel anger, guilt, or even sorrow right away. I felt a tremendous sense of relief that she was finally home safe. I sensed that she could see clearly now and walk, talk, sing, and be joyfully independent again. I felt peaceful knowing that I had held her hand as she left this world.

Bonnie goes on to say, "I felt a deep sense of freedom for us both. I no longer had to worry about her choking on her food or falling down and breaking a limb or having a stroke. I felt free to carry on with my life as I had known it before she came to live with us."

If you are struggling with guilt about having your freedom back or for feeling relieved about the end of your caregiving journey, perhaps Wendy Hill's teachings around handling death and dying from a healthy perspective will help:

> My boyfriend actually came to me in a dream and said, "We are given life to be happy and enjoy our lives. You're not. You're angry and sad because of me and my death. I need you to be happy. It is bothering me that you're not happy or enjoying your life, and I know it's because of me." He told me how hard it is for him to be at peace when I'm crying and so sad because of him. He went on to say, "Did you ever hurt someone and know that this person is crying because of you and you can't apologize or comfort them?" He said it's not easy to be enjoying the spirit

146

world when loved ones are miserable on the Earth. So, he said, "Every day you have here, you get to make all the choices to be enjoying life and you're not enjoying yourself."

PRACTICAL EXERCISE — HONOUR YOUR CAREGIVING ROLE

Journal about your caregiving experience, the positive and the negative. Write about the ups and downs, twists and turns, successes and failures. Be as thorough as possible. When you are done, have a ceremony and truly acknowledge yourself for being the best caregiver you could be with the tools, knowledge, and resources you had. Celebrate yourself and remember your loved one appreciated what you did for them and does not want you to remain trapped in guilt and regret. It is certain that they would not want you beating yourself up but instead would want you to live in freedom.

REFLECTIVE QUESTIONS

- How can you start truly enjoying your newfound freedom (without guilt and regret)?

- How can you honour your loved one by doing something special for yourself in their memory?

- Would your care recipient want you to be happy and go on living your life in peace? How could you move forward in peace and freedom to honour their wishes for you?

MAKE PEACE WITH THE PAST

It is quite possible you are feeling bad about certain aspects of your caregiving journey. The fact is, there is no such thing as a perfect caregiver. We've all done things we're not proud of and said or did hurtful things during our caregiving experience. As a result, it is not uncommon to feel guilty, ashamed, or angry with yourself for things you did or didn't do as a caregiver. While it is not healthy to focus on our mistakes, it can be helpful to reflect on them in order to reinterpret and/or release them. Forgiving ourselves is an important part of the grieving process. Without this, we continue to carry guilt and shame instead of the love and joy that we deserve.

PRACTICAL EXERCISE – FORGIVE YOURSELF

Think about at least three occasions where you felt guilty or had regrets related to your caregiving journey. Once you have them, close your eyes and imagine yourself standing in front of your loved one when they were still healthy. Have a conversation and say whatever you need to say to them that will allow you to release this regret and forgive yourself. Once the conversation is over, imagine yourself and your loved one putting these regretful events into a giant balloon. Once everything is in the balloon, imagine you and your loved one releasing it. Feel the lightness within you as you release these past regrets.

REFLECTIVE QUESTIONS

- If my child (or someone I love dearly) did the things I regret, would I be able to forgive them? Would I encourage them to forgive themselves?
- Can I give myself permission to forgive myself and move on with peace in my heart?
- In what ways would I feel empowered to go on with my life in a positive way if I were to truly forgive myself for certain aspects of my caregiving journey?

MAKE PEACE WITH THE NOW

Suffering is often a direct result of the difference between what is and what you want it to be. While you may not like your current reality, fighting it will only serve to prolong the agony. The most disempowering mantra you could possibly adopt is: I'll be happy when _____ (fill in the blank). The moment you embrace "what is" in the present moment is really the moment you find inner peace. What if you were to adopt the belief that everything is always working out for you, even when you don't see the bigger picture or understand the higher purpose? What if you could trust that the universe is giving you the exact experiences you need to fulfill your life's purpose? What if you could move forward from this experience with appreciation in your heart and joy in your soul knowing that the caregiving experience you had in its entirety, the positives and negatives, are what brought you to this exact point in time? The person you are right now in this exact moment is simply a collection of experiences. Therefore, it is important to acknowledge all of your experiences, all of your moments, and embrace *all* of who you are. In all of my efforts and all of my travels along my extensive search for inner peace, this is the only true key to happiness I have discovered.

PRACTICAL EXERCISE — INTEGRATE YOUR EXPERIENCE

If you had a magic wand, what experiences would you delete from your caregiving history (you can include your entire history if you wish to do deeper work)? Journal about these events in as much detail as you can, because these are the things you must reintegrate. Let me explain. If you think of yourself as a puzzle with a thousand pieces, and you cast away 200 of those pieces, you will never feel whole and complete. You will always be restlessly seeking happiness from external sources when actually you are seeking your own missing pieces. The same balloon exercise above can be used to make peace with these disowned experiences and parts of yourself.

REFLECTIVE QUESTIONS

- What if your caregiving experience was exactly what you needed for your growth and development?
- How has your caregiving experience changed your perspective on life?
- Can you find the deeper lessons and blessings in your caregiving experience?

RECONNECT AND REEVALUATE

It is completely normal to feel a little lost or like you don't know who you are any more — to be questioning and reevaluating your life as you try to redefine who you are as an individual — after your caregiving role. If your caregiver role started a long time ago, you may not remember who you were or what you enjoyed doing. Even if you do remember, it is almost certain you've come out of your caregiver experience a different person. Now you may be wondering, "Where do I go from here?" or "What do I do with my life now?"

Perhaps you lost touch with old friends or stopped engaging in the activities you used to enjoy. It is not unusual for caregivers to find themselves at a loss once they are free from their caregiving duties.

PRACTICAL EXERCISE — CREATE A NEW VISION

Lie down, close your eyes, and imagine your life one year from now. See yourself one year older and one year wiser. Reflect on how you want to spend your time and energy during the year following the end of your caregiving role.

REFLECTIVE QUESTIONS

- What areas of your life would you like to improve?

- What did you enjoy doing before your caregiving journey began? What do you enjoy doing now? What might you enjoy doing (activities you've thought of trying)?

- Who did you enjoy spending time with before your caregiving journey began? Who do you enjoy spending time with now? Who might you enjoy spending time with (people you are interested in getting to know better)?

TAKE CARE OF YOURSELF

Perhaps you have managed to stay connected with your friends, continued doing what you love to do, and kept yourself as a priority throughout your caregiving journey. However, I would venture to say that for most, this is not the case. Through my caregiving experience, I put myself on the back burner, and there was a huge cost to that. However, when my caregiving journey came to an end, I made a conscious decision to change my life and make myself a priority. I wanted my health and vitality back. I needed to reconnect with myself and rediscover the essence of me. At first, I didn't know how I was going to do it, but I started with a commitment of one hour a day of me time, even if it meant getting up a bit earlier in the morning. Starting wasn't easy, but I pushed through the first few weeks. Every day got easier and easier, and before I knew it, I was craving that "me time." It wasn't long before I noticed I was feeling healthier and stronger in body, mind, and spirit. I felt myself slowly regaining a sense of joy and freedom, starting with just a glimpse here and there. Eventually, I became more committed and disciplined about getting into an optimum state of wellness. I knew what it felt like to be at my lowest point, and I wanted to feel what it would be like to be at my highest. I wanted to meet the best version of *me*. If you are craving this too, complete the Self-Care Questionnaire (Appendix C) and follow these seven incredibly effective strategies:

1. Get a Coach

I won't harp on this one, because it was covered in the last chapter, but I will quote Einstein and say, "We can't solve problems by using the same kind of thinking we used when we created them." If you want a chance to be the best version of yourself, find someone who will help you get motivated and committed to yourself and who can give you the tools to keep your thoughts, feelings, and actions in alignment with the essence of who you are — your goals, your vision, your purpose, and your mission. A good coach is the best investment you can make. Remember, you are worth it!

2. Schedule Some Me Time

Schedule some "me time," even if it's just thirty minutes a day. Start taking some time every single day to do things that really energize you, and spend time with people who elevate your mood and your spirit.

3. Start the Day Right

Many rush out of bed in the morning (after hitting the snooze button three times) and get straight to worrying about what the day might bring. While worrying, they pound back a few cups of coffee, check emails, and try to figure out how they will meet all of the demands of the day. Instead of pressing the snooze button, take fifteen minutes before getting out of bed and start your day right by developing a morning routine that is conducive to a state of peace and happiness:

- Thank your higher power for giving you one more day on this planet. Be thankful that you woke up and have an opportunity to experience life again.

- Get in tune with your energy by using your awareness to scan every part of your body, starting at the top of your head. Relax each muscle as you scan it. Imagine the cells in your body dancing and visualize happy energy in your body.

- On a scale of 1 to 10, rate your energy level (1 being low and 10 being high). If your number is below 8, ask yourself what you can do to raise it.

- Set three priorities for the day that will contribute to increasing your energy and your state of happiness.

- Listen to a short self-affirmation script (perhaps one you created in the previous chapter).

- Look in the mirror for a full minute and check in with yourself. Ask yourself how you're doing. Ask what you can do to increase your energy and wellness. While looking in your own eyes, commit to being good to yourself today.

4. End the Day Right

Engaging in calming activities and turning electronics off at least thirty minutes before bed will do wonders for your mental and physical health. As much as it can be tempting to watch one more episode, read one more chapter, check one more website, or play another game before going to bed, resist the urge and instead create a bedtime routine that is conducive to a state of optimum wellness.

- Look in the mirror and check in with yourself. Ask yourself how you're doing. Ask whether you were good to yourself today. While looking in your own eyes, recommit to keeping yourself well.

- Listen to one of your self-affirmation scripts. Filling your mind with positive messages right before bed is one of the best ways to get your subconscious mind working for you.

- Breathe. It's hard to believe, but we often forget to breathe, or at least to breathe deeply. Take a moment before bed to take at least three deep breaths. Or you can try another effective breathing strategy ... simply breathe in for eight counts, hold your breath for four counts, and breathe out for seven counts. This breathing technique not only distracts your mind but also has a genuine calming effect on your nervous system.

- Get in tune with your energy by using your awareness to scan every part of your body, starting at the top of your head. Relax each muscle as you scan it.

- Put your worries away for the night. To do this, place a small box on your night stand. When a worry comes up, imagine yourself putting it in the box and remind yourself that it will be there in the morning. If you're a visual person, you may need to write your worries on a piece of paper and physically put it in the box. Once all of your problems have been put away, imagine a light switch in your brain and flick it off. If your mind wanders back, simply remind yourself that your problems are safely stowed away and do not give yourself permission to revisit them until morning.

- If you find yourself unable to sleep, instead of allowing your mind to go off in a million different directions and keep you awake at night, count backward from one hundred until you fall asleep. It is important to train your mind that the night is time to refresh, rejuvenate, and recharge.

5. Practice Gratitude

As Sandi Emdin explains in the **Caregiving Insights**, her palliative care training had awakened her to the certainty of death but also to the preciousness of life and snapped her out of taking her life for granted.

> On the rides home after training, I remember feeling grateful to be alive and thinking, over and over, "Thank you." I'd be thinking of how grateful I was to be healthy, to have a healthy husband, and healthy kids; how lucky I was to be a stay-at-home mom. This shift in thinking was new for me. I would have been much

more likely at the time to be complaining about the kids, my husband, or serious matters like having only one car. This new practice, new mindset, new attitude of gratitude, somehow left me feeling more joyful, more appreciative, and somehow lighter.

When I first started this gratitude practice over twenty years ago, I had a hard time coming up with just a few things to be grateful for, but now I can go on and on until I'm out of breath. It feels amazing every time. This lesson really changed my life. I learned when you feel grateful for what you have, you feel more happiness and joy. Up until then, I thought it was the other way around. I now practice thoughts of gratitude every day; when I first open my eyes, when I'm in the shower, at a traffic light, while I am cooking. It changes everything. Practicing a state of gratitude required more self-awareness than I was used to, yet so many gifts came from it. Ironically, this new awareness and gratitude for the gift of life came from weeks of talking about death. I had this new feeling of aliveness. I started to notice how much I complained, so I tried to count my blessings instead of the things I had to do when I got home. My usual mindset went something like this: "I have to pick up the kids, I have to get groceries, I have to gas up the car, I have to, I have to, I have to." This was not only exhausting, but it also sucked all the joy out of my day because I was focused on all the things I had to do. My mindset started shifting from thinking about all the things I had to do to the things I "got to do," because I could. I was alive. I was healthy. I still had time and energy to do things. It was only a minor shift in words yet such a major shift in thinking and feeling. I started thinking, I "get to" pick up the kids because I HAVE kids; I "get to" go grocery shopping because I have a car, money, and a family I love to feed. I "get to" cut the grass because I have a lawnmower and I know how to work it. This change in mindset was a seemingly small shift in thinking, yet it created a huge shift in the way I feel, keeping me in a daily state of gratitude for being alive.

The three small words "I get to" changed Sandi's life and can change yours too. Although it may be tempting to focus on the things that are going wrong throughout the day, resist the urge. Instead, start a gratitude practice and think about what you are grateful for. Remember, it is your choice whether you focus on the positive or the negative, and that choice will significantly impact how you feel.

6. Practice Mindfulness

Mindfulness is one of the most effective ways I have found to enhance my own personal sense of wellness. If you haven't already started a mindfulness practice, do yourself a huge favour and make a commitment to do so. Mindfulness can be done in one minute or less. Just take a moment to sit quietly, take three deep breaths, and whenever a thought comes up, notice it, detach from it, and bring your attention back to your breathing. You can repeat a mantra such as "I am here" over and over again. An even simpler practice is to simply commit to being fully present for a few minutes at a time. Watch and listen with your full attention. This is a great practice to commit to with your care recipient and is almost guaranteed to help you enjoy more moments with them.

7. Adopt a Healthy Lifestyle

Cutting down on sugar, caffeine, and alcohol can go a long way in helping you feel better. This, combined with eating whole foods, regular exercise, and getting adequate sleep (a minimum of seven hours per night), can immediately start improving your overall health and put you in an optimum state of wellness.

PRACTICAL EXERCISE — NEW PRESCRIPTION

Write several of the activities listed above on individual pieces of paper (small pieces). For example, "breathe," "be grateful," "exercise." Note you can be more specific and write "take three deep breaths," "write five things you are grateful for," "go for a fifteen-minute walk." Write at least ten activities, then fold each paper and place it in a Mason jar. When you are having a challenging moment, choose one from your jar as a reminder of things you can do to feel better. Think of it as your prescription bottle.

REFLECTIVE QUESTIONS

- What is your current quality of life on a scale of 1 to 10?
- What can you start doing immediately to enhance your quality of life?
- How committed are you to your own wellness?

CONCLUSION

In Dialectical Behaviour Therapy (DBT), there is a concept called Radical Acceptance, which basically means accepting reality, because fighting it only makes things more difficult and intensifies difficult emotional reactions. With this in mind, I will end this chapter with the wise words of Dr. Carole Tessier from her chapter, "Supporting End of Life Care," in the *Caregiving Insights*:

> People often pray or offer life compromises in hopes of getting a certain wish or outcome in life. An example is the parent who prays or offers a life full of sacrifices to save the life of their sick child, or even going further and negotiating their own life in exchange for their terminally ill child to be saved. When my three-year-old daughter was diagnosed with leukemia, I cried, I prayed, I begged, I negotiated, and I was ready to give anything for her to live. We may be so afraid or want things so desperately that we have a difficult time seeing the bigger picture. Another example is the person who prays to be loved by someone specific or who has difficulty accepting the end of a relationship. This reminds me of a Garth Brooks song titled "Unanswered Prayers" in which he tells the story about seeing an old high school flame, the girl he thought was The One, and how he had prayed to be with her. In the end, he thanked God for the gifts he had in his life and realized these gifts may not have been possible if his prayers had been answered. It speaks to how we can wish for something but later realize that there was another experience in store for us and we end up being thankful that our prayers weren't answered.
>
> Accepting happiness, or whatever is best for us and those around us, is not always what we think we want in the moment. It is about accepting some things are out of our control. Although I still wish my daughter and my family didn't have to go through these difficult few years, I have since been able to reflect on the growth we experienced both as individuals and as a family through our difficult ordeal with cancer. For me personally, it gave true meaning to Bob Marley's quote, "You

never know how strong you are until being strong is the only choice you have.

In my role as a caregiver I just have to accept that I cannot fix things, and the best I can do is support someone on their journey, whether it be at the beginning, at the end, or somewhere in between. Some days are harder than others, but I always try to remember to be grateful for being where I am meant to be and for helping people as best as I can. And for the times I struggle, I like to remember the quote that says, "Sometimes the best thing you can do is not think, not wonder, not imagine, not obsess. Just breathe and have faith that everything will work out for the best."

FINAL THOUGHTS

When my publisher asked me to write a book on caregiving, I said, Sure, no problem! I had spent my career as a caregiver, I was offering workshops on self-care, and I'd had the caregiving experience with my grandmother. Initially, I thought of writing this book from a professional perspective, because I didn't feel as though I had much to offer from my "failed" caregiving experience with my grandmother. However, in the days after agreeing to write this book, it strangely started writing itself. This has never happened to me before in all of my years as a writer. It turned out that writing this book allowed me to process my thoughts about my own caregiving journey at a deep, introspective level and to release old emotional baggage I didn't even realize I was carrying. It was truly cathartic, and I hope this book helps you do the same and perhaps avoid some of the "mistakes" I've made. And if you've already made them, make peace with yourself, because your loved one would want you to enjoy the rest of your life.

APPENDIX A

CAREGIVER CHECKLIST

As a caregiver, you will not only have to keep track of your own life but also someone else's. Therefore, in order to avoid becoming overwhelmed, take a full day (or two) to set up a system to manage your care recipient's information and plan for the future. You may be thinking, *I don't have time to do this*, but taking the time to get organized will not only make you feel more confident as a caregiver but will also save you time and energy in the long run because you will no longer waste time searching for information and worrying about how to handle certain situations. Please note that this checklist is general in nature, and some items may not apply, depending on your care recipient's needs and abilities. This checklist is not meant to replace medical, legal, or financial advice; contact your professional advisers for specific advice.

	DONE	TO-DO
Collect basic information	❏	❏
Organize medical information	❏	❏
Organize financial information	❏	❏
Develop an emergency plan	❏	❏
Develop a care plan	❏	❏
Advance Care planning	❏	❏

1. Collect basic information (place copies of the following into one folder labelled *General*):

   - Driver's license
   - Social insurance number
   - Passport
   - Usernames and passwords for social media accounts
   - Birth certificate
   - Marriage certificate
   - Military identifiers

2. Organize medical information (place copies of the following in a folder labelled *Medical*):

   - Benefits agreement/coverage
   - Health card
   - Health insurance cards
   - Doctors' names and contact numbers
   - Pharmacy name and phone number
   - Medical insurance (name of company, contact person, and phone number)

3. Organize financial information (place copies of the following in a folder labelled *Financial*):

   - Last three tax returns
   - Name of banks, bank account numbers, passwords/PIN, and phone number of bank contact person and/or financial planner
   - Usernames and passwords for accounts (credit cards, property taxes, heating, utilities, phone/TV/internet, etc.)
   - Information about bills, loans, and other debts and assets
   - Blank cheque
   - Pension agreement
   - House/property titles
   - Vehicle ownerships
   - Insurance policies

- Keys: safety deposit box, home safe, etc.
- Bank account numbers and access information (passwords, PIN numbers)

4. Develop an emergency care plan (insert the following information in a folder labelled *Emergency*):

- Prepare an emergency folder with the information needed in case of an unexpected trip to the hospital
- Telephone tree of emergency contacts (names of children, close friends, other relatives, secondary caregivers, etc.)
- Plan for pet care, if applicable

5. Develop a care plan (see table below):

- Learn about your loved one's illness and prognosis
- Identify your care recipient's current level of care and needs
- Assess activity levels — what can be done with and without help?
- Who can help with what and when?
- Discuss goals, needs, interests, likes, and dislikes
- Is the physical environment safe?
- Name and number of contact person from a local association related to your care recipient's illness and any other community resources that could be of assistance

CARE TEAM

Name	Relationship	Phone #	Emergency #	Email Address

Health Issues (illness, prognosis):

Concerns:

Risks (physical, financial, medical, etc.):

Goals:

Strengths and Interests:

Current Needs (refer to Chapter 1, *Caregiving Responsibilities* section):

Needs	Who Is Responsible?	When?

6. Advance care planning (insert the following information in a folder labelled *Advance Care*):

- Substitute decision-maker
- Power of attorney for personal care
- Power of attorney for finances
- Final directives
- DNR, if applicable
- Updated last will and testament
- Organ donor card

APPENDIX B

STRESS ASSESSMENT QUESTIONNAIRE

Stress can wreak havoc on our lives and make us feel miserable, exhausted, and sick. Strangely, we are not always aware when we are under stress, because our symptoms have become so familiar to us that we think they are normal. Then we look around and see so many others with the same symptoms, and we truly start to believe that this is just the way it is. So, if you're comparing notes with other caregivers, you may not be getting an accurate assessment. And when you no longer recognize your symptoms of stress, you are at great risk of burning out mentally, physically, emotionally, and spiritually.

Take this short twenty-question survey to help you evaluate how stress is impacting your life. Once you complete the questionnaire, your results will tell you how you are doing in terms of your overall stress level.

Please note that this survey is not intended to be a substitute for professional advice, diagnosis, or treatment.

FIND YOUR STRESS LEVEL BY TAKING THIS SURVEY:

Rate yourself HONESTLY using the following scale:

- Always
- Usually
- Sometimes
- Rarely
- Never

Note: Try NOT to answer with "sometimes" unless necessary. Use this answer mostly for questions that are not applicable to you. For example, if you do not have a job, answer questions about work with *Sometimes*.

In the past month, how frequently have you experienced the following symptoms:

1. I have difficulty falling asleep and/or wake up more than once during the night

2. I am lacking energy and motivation to do routine tasks

3. I am frequently ill and/or have medical problems

4. I take medication for anxiety, depression, or sleep

5. My mood is irritable and I am quick to anger

6. I feel disconnected from friends and family

7. I feel anxious and tense

8. I feel resentful toward my care recipient and/or life in general

9. I feel sad and hopeless

10. I feel insecure, worthless, or like I'm not good enough

11. I feel dissatisfied with my life

12. I don't feel appreciated

13. I have significant family problems

14. I worry constantly

15. I don't have enough time, especially for myself

16. I worry about the future

17. I feel overwhelmed

18. Even minor problems frustrate me

19. I don't get pleasure in things like I used to

20. I feel like I'm just surviving

ANSWER KEY

Give yourself points for every question answered as follows:

- Always = 5 points
- Usually = 4 points
- Sometimes = 3 points
- Rarely = 2 points
- Never = 1 point

RESULTS

Your scores are not meant to be used as a clinical assessment. Rather, the information is intended to provide you with a general overview of the level of stress you are experiencing in your life.

Over 60 — Emergency!

You have high scores on the stress survey. This indicates that there is high stress in several areas of your life that require your IMMEDIATE attention. The level of stress you are experiencing is not sustainable in the long-term and will likely result in serious problems. It is therefore recommended that you make significant and immediate adjustments to your lifestyle (diet, exercise, attitudes, relationships, etc.) and consult a health professional.

Between 40-60 — Average

Your score on the stress survey is in the average range. This indicates that there is either a high level of stress in one main area of your life or several areas that requires some attention. Although 'normal' levels of stress may not pose an immediate threat, in the long term it can become chronic and result in serious problems. Working on the choices and habits that are causing unnecessary stress in your life will make a big difference to your overall wellbeing.

Under 40 — Great News!

Your score on the stress survey suggests your stress levels are manageable in all or most areas of your life. You have high resilience, good ability to deal with stress, and you are a good role model for others. Keep doing what you're doing while at the same time making sure you're not trying too hard to avoid problems or shying away from challenges.

APPENDIX C

SELF-CARE QUESTIONNAIRE

	YES	NO
1. Do you have a coach, counsellor, or trusted friend to help keep you on track?	_____	_____
2. Do you take regular breaks from caregiving?	_____	_____
3. Are you breathing deeply and consciously?	_____	_____
4. Are you managing your stress effectively?	_____	_____
5. Do you have a regular gratitude practice?	_____	_____
6. Are you exercising regularly?	_____	_____
7. Are you making healthy food choices?	_____	_____
8. Are you sleeping well?	_____	_____
9. Are you making time for meditation and reflection?	_____	_____
10. Are you getting enough "me time"?	_____	_____

For the questions you answered "No" to, consider developing an action plan to make immediate positive changes in these areas.

ACKNOWLEDGEMENTS

I am deeply grateful to all of my family and friends who supported me on this journey. I thank each and every one of you for believing in me and encouraging me to reach my full potential.

Thank you Mom (Jo Somers) for all of your proofreading and editorial suggestions. I would like to express my deepest gratitude to Allister Thompson and Blue Moon Publishers.

A million thanks.

ABOUT THE AUTHOR

LISE LEBLANC, BA, MED., RP

Lise Leblanc has the experience and insight to make your caregiving journey a little lighter. As a registered psychotherapist, conflict resolution specialist and caregiver she has seen the impact that caregiving without personal care can wreak on all lives involved. Her personal lived experience has also shaped her useful perspectives. She was the main caregiver for her grandmother who had Alzheimer's disease when her grandfather died suddenly. Her own parents and siblings lived afar and she was working full time while raising her two young children. The experience has shaped her dedication to helping people take responsibility for the quality of their own lives at the same time as making space to support a conscious caregiving model.

Lise has a bachelor's degree in psychology and a master's degree in educational leadership, as well as several other therapeutic and mediation certifications. Along with the *Conscious Caregiving Guide Workbook* and *Caregiving Insights*, her mission in writing this *Conscious Caregiving Guide* is to give readers the knowledge, insight, and strategies to become more conscious caregivers.

NEXT CHAPTER PRESS

We create books that help people through life's transitions.

We all face changes, transitions, and life-altering experiences during the story of our life. From milestones to tragedies, some chapters are joyful and exciting, while others are sad and challenging.

If you are turning a page in your life, we hope our books will be a source of comfort, strength and inspiration. Written by people who have been through what you're experiencing or have helped others along a similar path, our books will help you move forward with experiences shared, lessons learned, and wisdom gained.

Everyone's story is written with many chapters, and we hope our books accompany you during this next stage of your life and help make it as meaningful as possible.

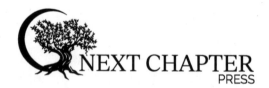

An Imprint of Blue Moon Publishers